Practical Problems in Dermatology

Second Edition

Practical Problems in Dermatology

Second Edition

Ronald Marks, FRCP, FRCPath
Professor of Dermatology
University of Wales College of Medicine
Cardiff, UK

MARTIN DUNITZ

To Hilary who encouraged me and thought the project worthwhile

© Ronald Marks, 1983, 1996

First published in the United Kingdom in 1983
by Martin Dunitz Limited Ltd
7–9 Pratt Street
London NW1 0AE

Reprinted and revised 1984
Reprinted 1985
Second edition 1996
Reprinted 1997

A CIP catalogue record for this book is available from the British Library

ISBN 1-85317-050-X

Composition by Scribe Design, Gillingham, Kent, UK
Printed and bound in Singapore by Kyodo Printing Pte Ltd

Contents

Introduction

Despite the fact that a family doctor can expect around 15 per cent of his or her consultations to be dermatological, skin diseases, though visible, are generally poorly understood by the nonspecialist. Their frequency and variety ensure that they are often a source of confusion to practitioners and all concerned with primary medical care. Is the rash catching? Will it get worse or rapidly go away? Will this or that treatment make it worse, make it better, or do nothing? These are just some of the questions that flood into the medical attendant's mind during examination. This book hopes to remove some of these uncertainties.

This is a pragmatic and practical book that assumes the reader knows little or no dermatology but wishes to improve the way that he or she copes with skin disorder. I have been guided by two major considerations in my choice of subject matter: the frequency with which a problem is encountered in general practice, and the severity of the distress it causes. I have covered some subjects in more detail than is found in most dermatological books for the very reason that they are dealt with so inadequately elsewhere. Inevitably this has meant concentrating on topics with a social flavour.

The book is not primarily intended for dermatologists, but I would be flattered if some of my colleagues read it. It contains little theory, is not intended to be comprehensive, and will only deal with the commoner conditions. However, I hope that there are some medical students and nurses who are tuned in to dermatology enough to want to read it.

If this book helps physicians to deal better with the problems of dermatological diagnosis and therapy they are likely to encounter regularly, and serves to dispel some of the myths and mystique associated with skin disorders, I shall be well satisfied.

Drug names

Throughout the text drugs are referred to by their generic and British trade names only.

PART ONE: GENERAL PROBLEMS

1

Infants' skin

BACKGROUND

Despite the smooth and vulnerable appearance of a baby's skin, it seems to be quite similar to adult skin when examined microscopically. All the anatomical structures are present and look complete. It is true that in some body sites some structures are much less well developed than in maturity – for example, in the infant hair follicles and sebaceous glands are tiny on most areas apart from the scalp. This is a reflection of the immaturity in sexual function and, as may be expected, there are other differences between infantile skin and the skin in maturity as far as function is concerned. The dermal connective tissue appears no different from that of an adult when histological sections are examined, but biochemically it is immature and much less tough mechanically.

There are important differences in heat regulation between infants' and adults' skin. This is due to the different area to body volume ratio, the skin's vascular reactivity and its ability to lose heat by sweating in infancy. The result is that body temperature regulation in infancy is far more subject to variation after relatively minor stimuli.

Differences between infant and adult skin

- **Epidermis and stratum corneum**
  No differences in structure, but stratum corneum may not be so tough in infants.
- **Dermis**
  Thickens progressively up to age of 20.
- **Hair**
  Tends to be finer and less dense on scalp in infants.
  Secondary sexual hair (axillae, pubis, beard area) starts to appear at puberty.
- **Sebum**
  Increased rate of secretion after puberty.
- **Sweat**
  Increased rate of secretion after puberty.
- **Pigmentation**
  Tends to increase till maturity.

It is often suggested that infantile skin presents less of a barrier to the penetration of substances applied to it. Interestingly, experiments have not confirmed this and any apparent susceptibility to intoxication from the application of materials topically seems to be due to the different surface-to-body volume ratio mentioned above.

NAPKIN DERMATITIS

Skin was not intended to withstand attack from a semisolid alkaline mixture of urine and faeces held in contact with the skin surface for two or three hours at a time. It is a marvellous tribute to the efficiency of the skin's structure that napkin dermatitis does not occur in 100 per cent of infants! Not only is buttock skin insulted by being bathed in this loathsome soup, but the barrier is often further compromised by the use of rough and abrasive materials to hold it in contact. Even worse, the social requirements of removing the inconveniences of infantile excretion from the gaze and nostrils of family and friends have encouraged the use of occlusive rubber or plastic pants which ensure

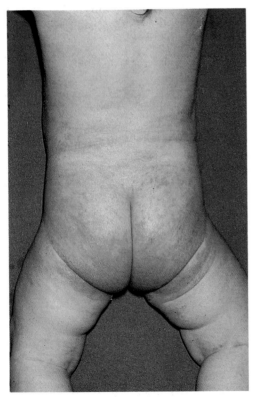

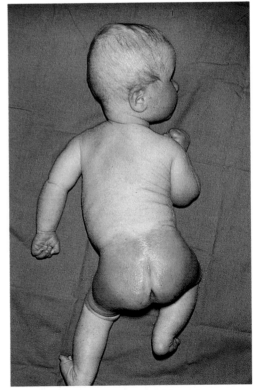

Mild napkin dermatitis. This degree of inflammation is not uncommon but is easily dealt with by changing the napkins more frequently and using emollients.

Moderately severe napkin dermatitis. Notice the sparing in the flexures, indicating that the sites of maximal involvement are those in intimate contact with the napkin.

that the skin becomes strongly saturated and its surface less efficient at withstanding attack. What about 'disposable nappies', you ask. Modern day 'disposables' are specially designed to soak up the urine but keep the skin/material interface dry and clean. They are much improved compared to the older products which seemed to encourage a dermatitis rather than prevent one.

Types of reaction

Irritative redness and scaling The commonest type of reaction to the irritation of napkins and their contents is the appearance of redness and scaling. Erosions sometimes appear, especially when there is a strong smell of ammonia and the faecal–urinary mixture is alkaline. The reaction may affect the whole of the napkin-covered area but is more usually localized to the convexities of the buttocks (the sites of maximum contact with the napkins) and only occasionally involves the flexures.

Dermatitic The reaction may be more dermatitic than irritative and here it tends to occur in a more haphazard manner in the napkin area, not being strictly confined to areas of maximal irritation. When dermatitic, the rash quite often spreads to involve other parts of the body – particularly the scalp and trunk and within the body folds. Curiously enough, when an infant has atopic dermatitis (see also pages 15–17) the napkin area is the one part of the skin that is spared.

Psoriatic Occasionally the rash in the napkin area is more like psoriasis: its margins are quite well defined, its colour is a dull, glazed red and there may even be large psoriasiform silvery scales. This so-called 'napkin psoriasis' also tends to spread to other parts of the skin surface, particularly the flexures and the face and scalp. Its relationship to proper psoriasis is still being debated but it is quite different in one respect – it responds quickly to treatment and rarely remains troublesome in childhood.

Moniliasis ('thrush') There has been a tendency to believe that napkin dermatitis is due to infection with *Candida albicans*. This belief stems from the ease with which this yeast-like micro-organism can be recovered from the napkin area. The real role of *Candida* is unclear and is likely to be of real significance only when the groin and internatal flexures are involved. Mostly it is a secondary invader or a contaminant.

Treatment

All the above varieties of napkin rash are due ultimately to the same thing – irritation from the napkin and its contents. It follows that treatment should be directed at reducing both the degree and time of contact between the damp, faecal covering and the skin surface. A brief chat with the mother about the gentle care of her beloved's rear end is essential. Explain that:

1. Rubber or plastic panties worn over the napkin are to be avoided.
2. If disposable napkins are to be used, use only the best.
3. Coarse towelling can also abrade the skin, so where possible smoother materials should be substituted.

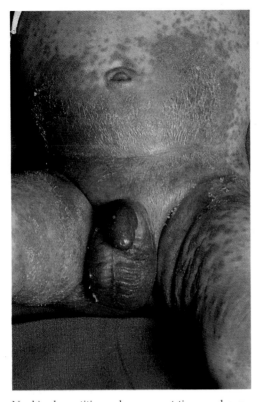

Napkin dermatitis can be severe at times and may spread well outside the napkin area. In this youngster the rash has spread to the abdomen and in fact there were affected areas on the arms and neck as well.

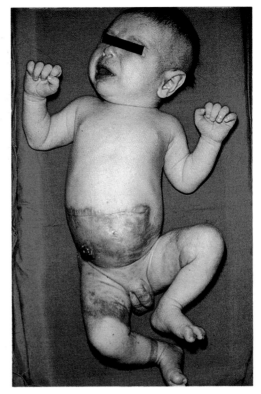

Napkin psoriasis. The relationship of this disorder to adult psoriasis is unknown. The affected area can look somewhat like psoriasis, with a well-defined edge and psoriasiform scaling. (This baby had recently undergone a bowel operation.)

4. Whatever the kind of napkin used, it has to be changed frequently!
5. When possible the infant should be kept for periods without any covering at all.

As mentioned above the yeast organism that causes thrush is more likely to be a secondary invader or a contaminant rather than a true pathogen. Consequently the use of preparations containing nystatin or other antifungal agents has only marginal value. The same holds for bacteria of various types and there is little to be gained from using the various antiseptic compounds promoted for this purpose. The inflamed area needs very little in the way of topical applications and will often improve spontaneously if care is taken over use of napkins. A reasonable plan is to start off with an emollient cleanser of some sort, and a bland emollient application some two or three times per day after cleansing. Powders do very little and can make matters worse by caking and clogging in the flexures and causing further irritation. If the rash is very red and angry, and quite widespread over the body, a little 1 per cent hydrocortisone application is in order. Stronger corticosteroids should not be used (see Chapter 27). They do no particular good

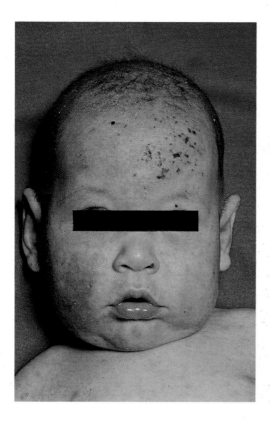

Typical atopic dermatitis affecting the face of a 7-month-old girl. This youngster's rash started at the age of 4 months. Areas behind the knees and on the arms were also involved.

in this situation and can cause a great deal of harm. There are cases recorded of infants who have had not only skin thinning but severe muscle wasting of the buttocks from the use of strong corticosteroids.

ATOPIC DERMATITIS

This begins between the third and sixth month in many infants but may start as early as 4 weeks of age or as late as 2 years old. The skin is generally rough and dry, and there are pink and scaling areas. Scratching and rubbing doesn't start till the child is about 6 months old, when scratch marks (excoriations) become evident. Continual rubbing and scratching produces a characteristic type of skin thickening in which there is exaggeration of skin surface markings, known as lichenification. The way that some affected babies scream at night and tear at their skin is very distressing to the parents and the disorder must be thought of as a familial problem. Localization to the typical flexural sites may occur some time after the onset, but even so the diagnosis is usually straightforward. Particularly helpful is a family history of asthma or hay fever or of someone else with atopic dermatitis. The napkin area is often spared, in contrast to most other similar rashes in infancy, while the face and neck are frequently involved. Eye rubbing due to the persistent irritation results in darkening of the periocular skin and the appearance of an intraorbital fold, called the Denny–Morgan fold. After the first year typical sites of involvement are the antecubital and popliteal fossae as well as the wrists and ankles. Extreme itchiness is also helpful diagnostically. Emollients, weak corticosteroids and reassurance are the mainstays of treatment (see Chapter 15).

OTHER FORMS OF DERMATITIS

Infants are also prone to transient attacks of scaling pink patches around the face or flexures. They usually resolve after a few weeks without vigorous treatment. Some claim they are related to adult seborrhoeic dermatitis (see Chapter 33).

CRADLE CAP

We do not know why cradle cap forms. The crumbly debris forms specifically in the first few weeks of life and is confined to the scalp. It seems to consist of ordinary desquamated skin cells and is an infant analogue of dandruff in adults. There does not seem to be any relationship to seborrhoeic dermatitis. We do know that it is a benign and self-limiting disorder of infants in the first few weeks or months of life. It may only be necessary to recommend the use of a mild detergent-based shampoo two or three times per week. If further action seems necessary arachis oil or aqueous cream, with or without 2 per cent salicylic acid, can be applied and then gently washed off with a baby shampoo or combed out.

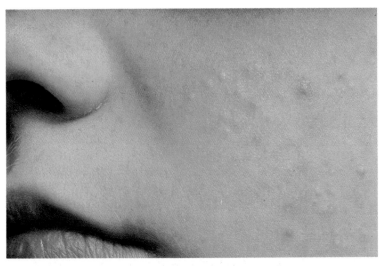

Infantile acne. Note there are many comedones and small papules on the cheeks of this child. The larger lesions seen in adolescents do not occur.

ACNE

Typical acne spots are quite commonly seen on the cheeks and forehead of infants. They are very uncommon on the trunk. As in adult acne the types of lesions seen include blackheads, pustules and small papules (see Chapter 21). Luckily, large inflamed papules and cysts and the consequent scarring are not seen. The acne spots usually disappear spontaneously after some weeks or months but some seem to persist and this may cause parental anxiety. Infantile acne tends to be transient in the first few weeks of life but more stubborn when the lesions develop later in the first 2 years. Mild topical treatments should be used – the weaker concentrations of tretinoin or benzoyl peroxide are suitable. The parents should be warned that, although effective, these agents can produce skin irritation and the frequency of application may have to be reduced.

BIRTHMARKS

Flat reddened patches are commonly seen on the back of the scalp in neonates, but most of these quickly disappear without treatment. They seem to represent some transient type of vascular malformation.

Port-wine stains over the side of the face, scalp and neck unfortunately do not disappear. These can be horribly disfiguring and cause much unhappiness. Youngsters with these abnormalities need to be seen by a paediatrician or dermatologist fairly early on in order to check whether there are neurological or ophthalmological components to the disorder. About the time they start school, affected children can be taught to use cosmetic camouflage by an expert, although in some less disfigured children it may be best to delay this until later.

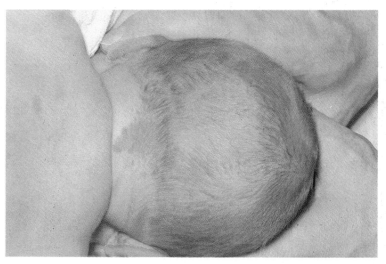

A port-wine stain on the back of the neck – popularly called a 'stork-mark'.

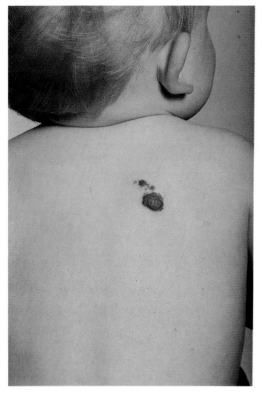

A typical strawberry naevus. Most of these lesions disappear at puberty.

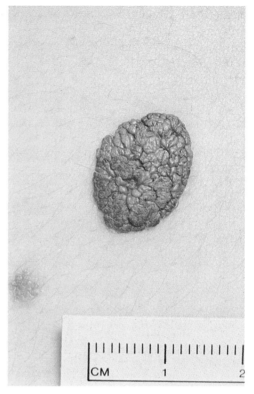

Moles usually appear during childhood but some are present at birth or shortly after. These are usually larger and uglier than the majority of moles.

Some of these vascular birthmarks can be much improved with laser beam treatment. Not all can be helped in this way. Use of the right equipment is of fundamental importance, as are the skill and experience of the operator. Different lasers are required for different tasks and the concentration of resources needed dictates that there are relatively few centres that can offer the necessary treatment.

Luckily the large and deep cavernous type of vascular birthmark is quite uncommon. Some of these disappear, but some do not and need attention from a plastic surgeon.

Strawberry birthmarks differ in that they are localized, raised, and often lobulated – just like strawberries. The large majority of these lesions spontaneously disappear in late childhood, although sometimes they ulcerate and then require dressing and occasionally other types of specialist treatment. Rarely, some cause mechanical problems because of their size.

MOLES

Ordinary moles (naevi) do not usually appear before the early school years, but there are some moles that are congenital and are present from birth or shortly thereafter. Most of these are trivial and not disfiguring. However there are some, luckily rare, that are dreadfully deforming. Because they are often distributed over an entire segment of the trunk they have come to be known as 'bathing-trunk' or 'cape' naevi. Surgical removal is usually out of the question, although some of the smaller ones may be improved by surgery or laser treatment. A small proportion become malignant in later life, so that regular follow-up of these unfortunate patients is advisable.

PRACTICAL POINTS

- **Napkin dermatitis**
  1. All types can usually be controlled by frequent changes of napkins and the use of absorbent and non-occlusive materials.
  2. Bland emollient applications and cleansers are helpful.
  3. In severe cases a little 1 per cent hydrocortisone may be required.
  4. Do not prescribe antifungal or antiseptic agents, or medium or strong corticosteroid applications, or recommend talcum powders.
- **Atopic dermatitis**
  1. Diagnostic pointers:
     –Rough, dry skin
     –Pink, scaling scratched areas
     –Family history of atopy
     –Absence of inflammation in the napkin area
     –Involvement of face and neck
     –Extreme itchiness.
  2. Treatment:
     –Emollients
     –Weak corticosteroids
     –Reassurance.
- **Cradle cap**
  1. In most cases regular use of a mild, detergent-based shampoo will clear the condition.
  2. If not, arachis oil or aqueous cream, with or without 2 per cent salicylic acid, may be successful.
- **Acne**
  In infants this condition usually clears spontaneously, and so requires no treatment.
- **Birthmarks**
  1. Infants with extensive port-wine stains should be checked early for neurological and ophthalmological disorders by a specialist.
  2. Strawberry birthmarks generally disappear spontaneously and require no treatment.
- **Moles**
  Infants with 'bathing-trunk' or 'cape' naevi require regular follow-up.

2
Skin disease in schoolchildren

BACKGROUND

The decision to exclude a child from school is often taken too lightly. Many youngsters prefer to be uncomfortable and at school rather than slightly less uncomfortable but bored at home.

The issues are very different from those with an adult and his work (see Chapter 5). Acceptance by the peer group is of particular importance to children. They also tend to be both more sensitive than adults to appearing different, and yet more capable of adapting to disability. Children are also capable of the most appalling cruelty to their classmates and there is little more destructive to the evolution of a child's confidence than a gang of young thugs perpetually chanting 'Scabby' or 'Poxy'. The factors to be considered include the following:

1. The physical and functional ability of the child with the skin disorder to continue at school.
2. The possible aggravation of the skin disorder by the 'trauma' of school attendance.
3. The educational and/or emotional problems likely to arise in the child by his or her exclusion.
4. The problems likely to arise in the household by keeping the child at home.
5. The possibility of transmission of the disorder to schoolmates.

Familiarity with the family and insight into the fears and resistance of the youngster involved will help in reaching the most appropriate decision as to when, if, and for how long a child should be away from school. There is obviously much less of a problem with diseases that are either spontaneously short-lived or easily cleared with treatments. Particular problems arise with warts, ringworm and lice. The latter two may be less difficult because it is relatively easy to remove the problem. Warts – particularly plantar warts – cause problems but it seems illogical to prevent children swimming because of them as there is so much wart virus around anyway.

IMPETIGO

Impetigo is diagnosed as a weeping, golden, crusted eruption on the face, limbs and trunk. When treated with systemic antibiotics and local bathing, it should cease to be a problem

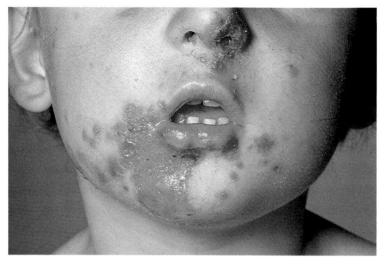

Quite severe impetigo in child attending infants' school. At this stage, with crusts and exudation, the lesions are infectious.

within a week. As this is easily transmitted to other children by contact, the child should not attend school while there is any crusting or ooziness about the lesions. Failure to respond to treatment may mean either that the condition is not impetigo but another disorder, such as herpes or eczema, or that the treatment has not been used.

SCALP RINGWORM

Scalp ringworm always causes a furore. Its prewar reputation lives on and strikes fear among parents and school staff alike. In reality there should not be much of a problem these days, providing that the disorder is recognized quickly. It is diagnosed as a localized, inflamed scaling area with hair loss and broken hair. After the diagnosis has been confirmed the child should be kept away from school and a search mounted among all the pupils for others with the infection. It is important to remember that in many countries scalp ringworm is a notifiable disorder.

It responds readily to oral griseofulvin (Fulcin, Grisovin), ketoconazole (Nizoral) or terbinafine (Lamisil) and providing that the infected hair is removed and the spores inactivated the child can return to school after three or four weeks. The disorder is usually caught from other pupils, and for this reason the local community physicians should visit the school in which an outbreak has occurred to examine the other children and take specimens for culture.

BODY RINGWORM

This type of ringworm may be caused by either animal or human species of ringworm fungus. It is probably best to prevent the infected child from participating in sports

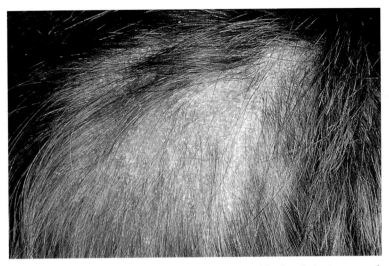

Ringworm of the scalp. There is some loss of hair and broken hairs in areas of the scalp. The skin of the scalp shows some scaling. At this stage the child is infectious.

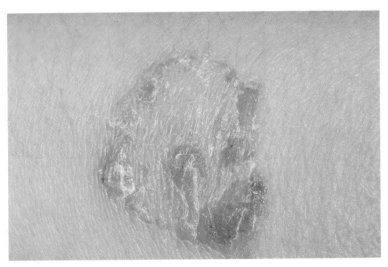

Ringworm of the trunk. The angry, raised, red border indicates that the disease is still active and infectious.

requiring communal bathing and changing facilities or likely to involve body contact while the infection is present. When antifungal treatment has been applied for around two weeks the affected areas should be flat and nonscaling, and then normal activities can be resumed. There does not seem to be any good reason for keeping the young patient away from school with ringworm infection of any site other than the scalp.

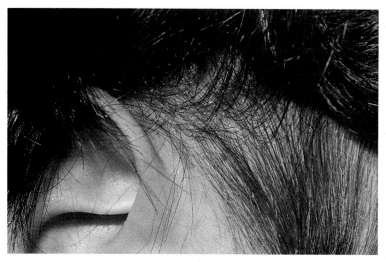

Child with infectious ringworm of the face.

'Athlete's foot'

What is frequently called 'athlete's foot' is due to a fungus infection in only about one quarter of those with scaling and maceration between the toes, ie, toe cleft intertrigo. In the rest it is due to a hotch-potch of causes including *Candida*, erythrasma, bacterial infection and just poor hygiene in those with overlapping toes. In these instances advice should be given on simple foot hygiene. If necessary a simple antimicrobial cream or lotion can also be prescribed – creams containing povidone-iodine or miconazole, for example.

SCABIES

Children generally acquire this disease from another member of the family and it doesn't seem to spread much within a school.

Treatment of scabies is dealt with on page 153 but some points need emphasis here. Treatment must be adequate, that is, the instructions that the entire body should be treated (save the face) must be obeyed. Treatment must be given for the entire family (that is, all those living together under one roof) and it should be checked that they apply it at the same time. After the initial mite-killing treatment – benzyl benzoate (Ascabiol), lindane (Quellada, Lorexane) or permethrin (Lyclear) – the child can return to school but he or she should carry a note from the practitioner explaining that the itch may well persist for two weeks or more but that the child is no longer contagious. Care should be taken with very young infants as application of the treatment causes considerable skin irritation in many cases.

LICE

There is currently an epidemic of head lice in children in Great Britain. Pediculus capitis has proved a successful social climber and now infests the heads of middle-class children

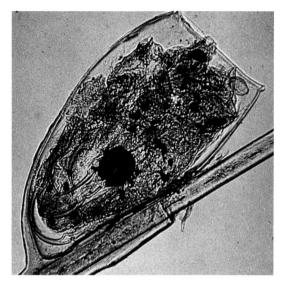

Close-up view of nit, showing immature form within.

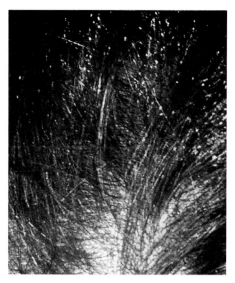

Nits visible on the hair at the nape of the neck in a young woman.

as frequently as those from less well-to-do homes. Pediculosis always causes shame and disgust in the affected family and alarm at school. In point of fact the infestation is (as far as we know) quite benign and apart from some itch, and perhaps infected scratches or mild dermatitis, causes no serious harm.

The diagnosis is often made by the school nurse who discovers the white eggs (nits) stuck to the shafts of the hair, although grandmothers are also known for their diagnostic acumen with this disorder.

A shorter hair style and adequate treatment – malathion (Derbac, Prioderm) – will deal with the problem (see page 152). The affected child should be kept away from school until the treatment has been given and no live lice or viable nits can be identified.

With the older remedies treatment must be given again after four weeks, in order to kill off any lice that emerge from any nits that remain behind. As many of the lice now infesting scalps around the Western world are resistant to these treatments it is better to prescribe the newer compounds.

Body lice are mainly seen in vagrants and in times of war and famine and are uncommon in children. Pubic lice are quite common in adults, but as children don't have much pubic hair and the disorder in adults is primarily due to venereal contact this infestation is rarely seen in this age group.

WARTS

Warts are due to virus infection of the epidermis and are contagious. The viruses responsible are different antigenic types of human papilloma virus. Warts are among the commonest of disorders and luckily rarely cause any significant threat to health. However, they are regarded as ugly and excite the usual distaste and revulsion associated with any disorder of the skin. Consequently they elicit a variety of illogical responses from teachers and local authorities, including the banning of children with plantar warts from swimming baths and from the gymnasium. For every visible plantar wart there must be many more that are not seen and exclusion seems a highly impractical way of preventing the spread of this disorder. It seems even more illogical when no attempt is made to prevent children who have had gastrointestinal or respiratory infections from swimming. In my view the obvious benefits that result from communal exercise far outweigh the minor hazards of wart infection, bearing in mind that these lesions are self-limiting and do not require heroic efforts at removal. They are anyway notoriously stubborn in resisting treatment (see Chapter 22).

ATOPIC DERMATITIS

Background

Atopic dermatitis is predominantly a disease of infancy and childhood and is an important cause of disability for children of school age (see also Chapter 15). Most dermatologists have the impression that children with atopic dermatitis tend to be more

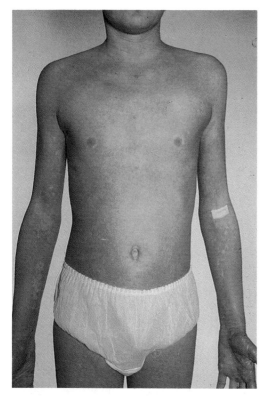

Persistent itching and soreness made this boy's atopic dermatitis very troublesome for him. It made school attendance extremely trying.

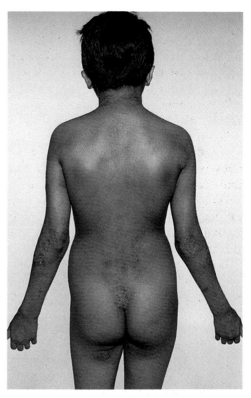

Extensive atopic dermatitis affecting the trunk, arms and thighs in a schoolboy. Many of the patches are thickened due to persistent rubbing and scratching.

intelligent than average and strongly motivated to school work and success. They also believe that these children are often tense and emotionally brittle. While there is little formal evidence derived from clinical practice to support these conclusions, my own clinical experience suggests that there may be some substance to them. Of course this is a real chicken-and-egg question. The association between these personality features and the skin disease may arise from the physical stress of the disease itself rather than the other way round, or they may even be directly unrelated, but linked genetically. There is, however, some evidence that atopic children are shorter in height than normal and this may affect their sporting interests at school and attitudes to them from their teachers and classmates. This shortness in stature could be due to the use of topical corticosteroids and the effects of the absorbed component of the applied steroids on the growth process. It is, however, more likely to be the result of the effects of the persistent emotional disturbance caused by the discomfort of itching and loss of sleep.

School attendance

The persistent itch caused by atopic dermatitis results in sleepless nights, soreness, infection and further inflammation of the skin (see also Chapter 17). It also produces parental anxiety, and a feeling of isolation for the child at school. The disorder is often at its worst in those years at school (9 to 16) when there is most to be gained from regular attendance and most emphasis is placed on educational achievement.

When the disorder affects the whole body, as unfortunately it frequently does, there is very little choice but to keep the child away from school. Apart from the difficulties of listening while itching mercilessly and the physical discomforts of moving around in a boisterous school environment when the skin is sore and sticking to the clothes, there is the real hazard of skin infection. Atopics are curiously prone to develop infections such as generalized herpes simplex and staphylococcal and streptococcal infection, and can be quite ill with these complications.

In many instances, when the disorder has flared and there is widespread involvement the child may need to be admitted to hospital because of the severity of local pain and discomfort as well as the pyrexia and the general unwellness if there is an infection. It is possible that the removal of the child from the antigens of his or her usual environment will also aid the process of resolution.

There are a few residential schools that are specially geared to the treatment of this type of chronic disability and provide a protected environment. They are suitable for the most severely affected children but luckily most sufferers from atopic dermatitis can battle through without leaving home.

The practitioner's role

Clearly, sufferers from atopic dermatitis deserve great sympathy. Part of the practitioner's task is to relieve the symptoms and remove or ameliorate the circumstances that aggravate the disease. The other major role to be played by the practitioner is that of education about the disease. The doctor should ensure that the family and the school staff know enough about the disease to support and protect the child during periods of intense discomfort. They should also be told the natural history of the disease and the complications that may occur. Usually, the disease will gradually improve through childhood and adolescence. However, in a small proportion (perhaps 2 or 3 per cent) it seems to be a lifelong disease.

Treatments

One or two more details of treatment are important in relationship to schooling.

Antihistamines Chlorpheniramine (Piriton), promethazine hydrochloride (Phenergan) and trimeprazine (Vallergan) are often prescribed to be taken in the evenings to calm the irritation and promote sleep at night. Unfortunately they are not always successful in these therapeutic aims and often give the child a 'hangover' in the mornings. If there is little or no beneficial effect they are best stopped or changed to a non-sedating antihistamine such as terfenadine (Triludan). It has to be said that there is very little evidence that any antihistamine has much of a role in damping down eczema.

Bandaging If the wrists, ankles and knees are very sore then they can be dressed at night with whatever topical agent is being prescribed, and covered by tubular bandages. It is probably unwise to dress them this way in the mornings because the child will arrive at school looking like an Egyptian mummy – the bandages only serve to emphasize the child's feeling of being different and will almost certainly drop off by midmorning!

Psychiatric consultation As mentioned above, atopic dermatitis seems to cause more parental anxiety than most other skin disorders. Family tensions grow and vicious circles become established. Under these circumstances it may be helpful to obtain the opinion of a psychiatrist who specializes in this type of family disturbance. They can often provide helpful advice and support the family through the problems that inevitably occur in this disorder.

PSORIASIS

Psoriasis is not common in childhood and when it does occur it is luckily not often severe. When severe and generalized psoriasis develops in young children the condition

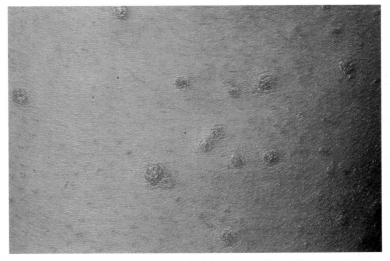

Guttate psoriasis. The individual lesions are quite small and do not tend to coalesce in the same way as in the adult disease. More frequently than not the condition starts after streptococcal tonsillitis.

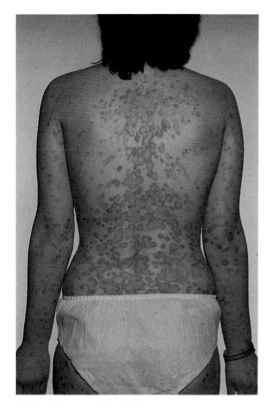

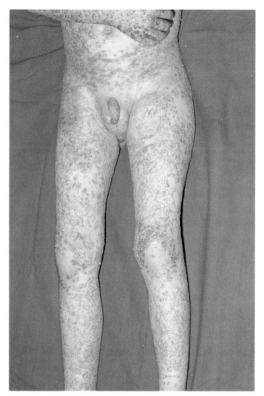

Quite widespread 'small-plaque' psoriasis in a 16-year-old. The lesions were not in visible areas and she found she could cope with school quite well.

Severe pustular psoriasis in a 7-year-old boy. The boy was affected suddenly and was generally very unwell and had a fever. Clearly school was impossible until the condition was cleared.

tends to be stubborn and difficult to treat. Guttate psoriasis may occur after a streptococcal throat infection in youngsters, but generally has a much better outlook than the adult plaque-type psoriasis. It should not interfere with schooling. If persistent psoriasis does occur during school years, care must be taken that the child is not given a 'leper' complex. Once again, careful explanation to parents and teachers is necessary. If the patches of psoriasis are quite widespread but not visible there is no real reason why the child should not continue at school and receive treatment at home (see Chapter 19). If it is generalized or the disorder occurs extensively over the arms or legs then it is kinder to try to arrange a period of in-patient treatment for the child.

Generalized pustular psoriasis is rare during childhood; where it does occur the child will need specialized care and school attendance will not be possible while the disease is active.

PRACTICAL POINTS

- **Impetigo**
This is quickly cleared with systemic antibiotics.
- **Scalp ringworm**
Responds well to griseofulvin (Fulcin, Grisovin) ketoconazole (Nizoral) or terbinafine (Lamisil) by mouth.
- **Body ringworm**
Takes around two to three weeks to clear with antifungal agents.
- **Scabies**
Treatment must be given for the entire family and all cohabitees and consorts.
- **Head lice**
Now usually resistant to older remedies, so more modern compounds such as malathion should be prescribed.
- **Warts**
In schoolchildren these are usually self-limiting and often resistant to treatment. If initial treatment is unsuccessful, warts are best left alone.
- **Atopic dermatitis**
If the whole body is affected the child should be kept away from school.
Emollient applications and bath oils are helpful.
Tubular bandaging is really only helpful at night.
Weak topical corticosteroids usually suffice to control the disease. Systemic antibiotics help many patients during acute flares of the disease – even in the absence of obvious signs of infection.
Systemic antihistamines should be used with care to avoid 'hangover' effect in mornings.
- **Psoriasis**
Not generally as severe a problem in schoolchildren as it is in adults.

3

Skin disease in pregnancy

NORMAL SKIN CHANGES

Marked changes take place in the skin during normal pregnancy. These should be recognized so as not to confuse them with disease.

Pigmentation

The skin becomes more darkly pigmented all over, but pigmentation in some sites is particularly marked. The darker the normal skin colour, the more marked this alteration is. The midline of the abdomen may darken and this feature is then known as the linea nigra. The nipples and areolae also darken. A curious pattern of uniform pigmentation may occur in certain areas of the face. The cheeks, central zone of the forehead, the

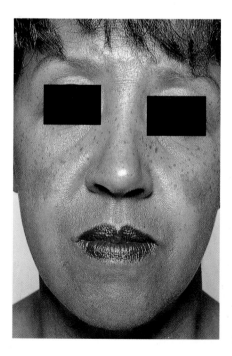

Chloasma (melasma). This is sometimes called the 'mask of pregnancy'. Pigmentation develops symmetrically over the face on either cheek, forehead and chin.

periocular areas, chin and temple skin may become pigmented to give a mask-like appearance – the so-called 'mask of pregnancy', sometimes known as chloasma. The pigmentation decreases after pregnancy but may take some months to do so and even then may never revert to exactly the same depth of colour present before pregnancy.

If advice is sought about this type of pigmentation during pregnancy, firm reassurance is the order of the day. If the woman is perturbed about her appearance and won't wait to see how much it improves after delivery then she should see a cosmetician (many large hospitals have one attached to the dermatology department). If there is still a problem some months after, then she should see a dermatologist. Although the pigmented areas are not easy to lighten there are some preparations, containing monobenzylether/hydroquinone, tretinoin (Retin A) or azelaic acid (Skinoren), for example, which are reputedly helpful, but which may require many months of use before the desired effects are seen.

Stretch marks

The skin of the lower abdomen, thighs and sometimes breasts may develop 'stretch marks', or striae gravidarum. These linear, red-purplish areas result from the stretching of the skin at the above sites in conjunction with the physiological hypercortisonism that occurs during pregnancy. Some striae are also seen during puberty, and in Cushing's

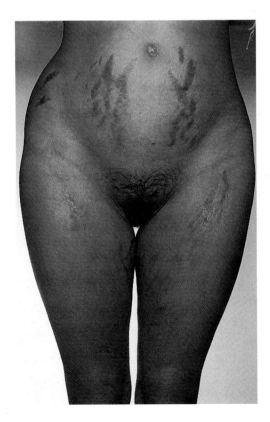

Striae distensae. These stretch marks develop over the abdomen and thighs mainly during pregnancy. They may also be seen around the breasts and on the upper arms. Although generally symptomless, their appearance causes distress.

syndrome many broad stretch marks are noted. They also appear during treatment with steroids, either by mouth or topically. Their anatomical basis appears to be the rupture of the dermal elastic fibres and this explains their irreversible nature. Although permanent in the sense that the skin in these lesions is never completely normal, they do contract down eventually to much less obvious, thin, whitish scars. Unfortunately there are no prophylactic measures that can prevent the marks and neither are there any effective treatments for them once present. There are preparations promoted to these ends but evidence for their effectiveness is lacking.

Other changes

The skin may be markedly greasier during pregnancy, particularly in the last trimester. Hair growth is not normally much altered, although pregnant women quite often complain that their hair is much less manageable at this time. A few weeks after delivery it is quite common for women to notice an increased loss of scalp hair. This is known as 'telogen effluvium'. It is a temporary and not usually very extensive loss. If shed telogen hairs are examined a small knob can be seen at one end instead of the usual long white collar on plucked hairs. This is supposedly due to the trauma of delivery throwing all the hair follicles simultaneously into the telogen or resting phase of the hair cycle.

Normal skin changes during pregnancy

- **Pigmentation**
  –Generalized
  –Midline of the abdomen
  –Nipples and areolae
  –'Mask of pregnancy'
- **Stretch marks**
  –Lower abdomen
  –Thighs
  –Breasts
- **Increased sebum secretion rate**

SKIN DISORDERS DURING PREGNANCY

Eczema and psoriasis

These disorders do not behave in any special way during pregnancy and there is no reason for a women with them to avoid pregnancy. If anything, they tend to improve at this time, and this may be due to the physiological hypercortisonism mentioned before. Any systemic therapy for either disorder must be stopped because of the danger of producing fetal abnormalities. Special care must be taken with the retinoid drugs etretinate (Tigason) and acitretin (Neotigason) as the risk of tetragenicity with these drugs is high and persists for up to two years after stopping either of these drugs.

Acne and rosacea

Acne may become somewhat more inflamed during pregnancy but this is not a regular occurrence. Systemic antibiotics should not be given – if a patient is receiving these, they must be stopped immediately if there is any suspicion of pregnancy. The risk of serious harm to the fetus varies with the antibiotics in question, but any risk on account of treatment for acne is unacceptable.

The same applies to rosacea, which usually responds so well to oral tetracycline. If treatment is required it may be permissible to use topical tetracycline or topical metronidazole: a small amount may be absorbed but if restricted to the face it is unlikely that enough will be absorbed to cause any harm.

Infective disorders

Of course, rubella is well known as a hazard to pregnancy. If the infection occurs during the vital first three months, there is a high risk of fetal abnormality.

Thrush (candidiasis or moniliasis) occurs more frequently in pregnant women and may occur in the groin and perioral areas and under the breasts as well as in the vagina. It causes considerable discomfort and itchiness, and patients should be referred to a specialist for treatment.

Chickenpox in the first three months may cause fetal abnormalities but in the last few weeks may give rise to intranatal chickenpox with the appearance of chickenpox vesicles on the skin of the fetus.

As far as is known, herpes genitalis in pregnancy does not cause fetal problems or alter the course of the pregnancy. However, natural delivery is best avoided during an attack of herpes genitalis and many obstetricians advise Caesarean section in these circumstances.

Pregnant women should be advised to avoid contact with known cases of all the above diseases.

Itchy rashes

For reasons we do not understand, the skin seems to be prone to irritation of many kinds during pregnancy. The stretch marks may become uncomfortably itchy in the later stages of pregnancy and the vulval area can also be affected by this embarrassing symptom for no very obvious reason. Generalized pruritus is also occasionally seen without obvious skin disorder.

Itchy rashes occur – particularly in the last three months of pregnancy. They are often widely distributed over the trunk and upper limbs and, because of their annoying itchiness, cause a lot of discomfort. The rashes can be urticaria-like or measles-like. Occasionally they develop tiny vesicles.

There is also a rare blistering disorder seen in the last few weeks or days of pregnancy (or even a few days post partum) known as herpes gestationis (also known as pemphigoid gestationis). This has nothing to do with herpes simplex or herpes zoster, and as far as we know is not caused by a virus. It may, however, be an indication for Caesarean section and can recur in subsequent pregnancies. It may even recur if the contraceptive pill is administered. Very little is known about the cause of these disorders, although in recent years there has been some advance in our understanding of the immunopathology of the rare herpes gestationis.

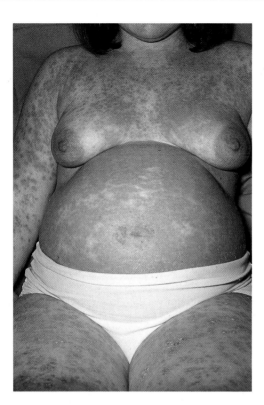

Itchy rashes in pregnancy are fairly common. This pregnant women's eruption developed at the beginning of the third trimester. It came on quite suddenly and was extremely itchy.

Luckily these rashes usually improve spontaneously a few days after delivery and are not associated with any other complication of pregnancy or fetal abnormality, although one type is said to be associated with a pre-eclamptic toxaemia. As mentioned above, some of these disorders may recur in subsequent pregnancies. When they cause intolerable itching it may be difficult to do much other than give some relief. Mentholated oily calamine lotion may also help relieve the itchiness. Potent sedatives and antihistamines are best avoided for fear of causing harm to the fetus.

PRACTICAL POINTS

- The patient should be reassured that the skin pigmentation associated with pregnancy will largely disappear after delivery; if this does not happen, she should be referred to a cosmetician.
- There are no effective prophylactics or treatments for stretch marks.
- Systemic treatments for any skin disease should be discontinued during pregnancy.
- Bland emollients or mentholated oily calamine lotion may help to relieve itching caused by rashes.

4
Problems concerning the inheritance of skin disease

BACKGROUND

There are few more delicate topics that a patient can introduce during a consultation than the possibility of the inheritance of his or her disorder. Honesty, tact and sympathy are needed. Many of the questions that are asked about inheritance of skin disease can be answered easily and reassuringly by the practitioner. Other questions require expert knowledge and possibly laboratory tests and should be left for the specialist to answer. Departments of medical genetics have a special and important role in this area.

PSORIASIS AND ATOPIC DERMATITIS

Psoriasis and atopic dermatitis are common diseases and most sufferers have heard that they run in families. In neither disease is it possible to state categorically the exact degree of risk of the condition being inherited. All that can be done is to discuss the chances of inheritance with the questioner in a broad, general way. With both disorders, if one parent is affected there is about a 20–30 per cent chance of a child eventually suffering from the parental disorder. If both parents are affected the risk is increased to about 50 per cent.

ICHTHYOSES

The generalized dry-scaling skin disorders known as the ichthyoses are genetically determined but the exact type of inheritance varies between different ichthyotic disorders. The only feature that they have in common is that there is some biochemical abnormality in the way that horn is formed and ultimately shed from the surface. As distinction between the different types depends on the clinical features these will be described briefly here.

Common ichthyosis

The commonest type is the least severe and is inherited as an autosomal dominant characteristic so that if one parent has the disorder, approximately half of the children

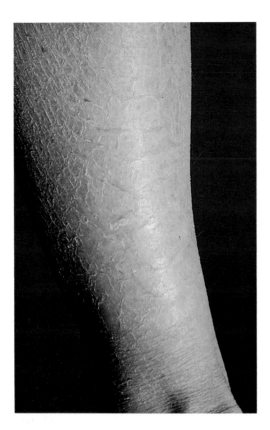

Typical autosomal dominant ichthyosis (ichthyosis vulgaris). The skin is dry and scaling.

will be affected. The condition is obvious shortly after birth and becomes more prominent later in life. The hallmark of the condition is scaling – the individual scales tend to be large, dingy grey or light brown, and shield-like in shape. Although the condition is generalized, the face and flexural areas tend to be spared.

Sex-linked ichthyosis

This is a similar condition to common ichthyosis but is inherited as a sex-linked disorder. This condition tends to be more severe – the scales are larger and more prominent and there is less sparing of the flexures. It is inherited as an X-linked recessive feature, that is, the condition is carried by women but only develops in males. There will be no affected male children if the father is affected, but girls from the union will be carriers and their sons may be affected. Special laboratory tests for diagnosing this condition have been developed and are available in some larger centres. These depend either on detecting an underlying enzyme defect – namely, steroid sulphatase deficiency – or on the results of its defective action. In the former kind of test, cultures of fibroblasts, epidermal cells or lymphocytes are set up and tested for their ability to split sterol esters. The latter type of test is less time-consuming and somewhat less technically demanding. The

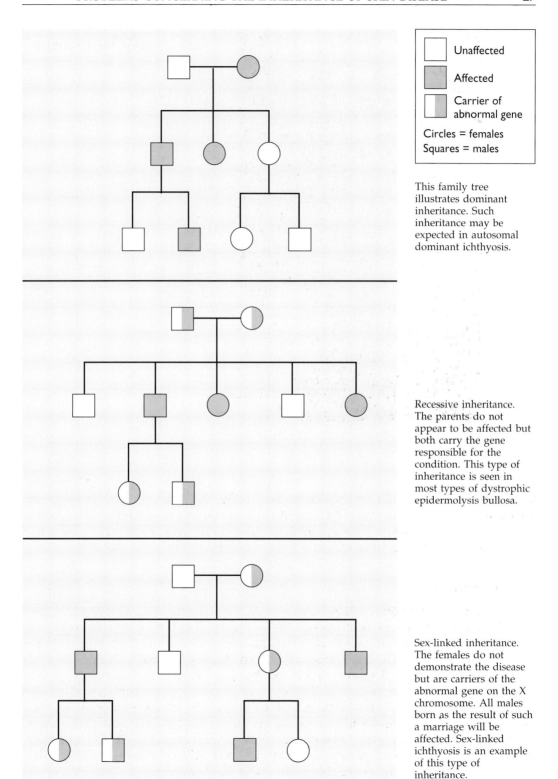

☐	Unaffected
▨	Affected
◧	Carrier of abnormal gene

Circles = females
Squares = males

This family tree illustrates dominant inheritance. Such inheritance may be expected in autosomal dominant ichthyosis.

Recessive inheritance. The parents do not appear to be affected but both carry the gene responsible for the condition. This type of inheritance is seen in most types of dystrophic epidermolysis bullosa.

Sex-linked inheritance. The females do not demonstrate the disease but are carriers of the abnormal gene on the X chromosome. All males born as the result of such a marriage will be affected. Sex-linked ichthyosis is an example of this type of inheritance.

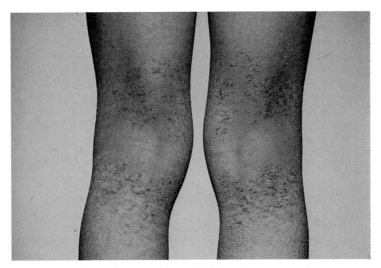

Sex-linked ichthyosis. This condition, which is only seen in males, is more severe than autosomal dominant ichthyosis, and the scales tend to be darker. Notice the sparing of the flexures. The gene for sex-linked ichthyosis is carried by the female but the disorder is only manifested in males.

determination of the ratio of free to esterified cholesterol in the stratum corneum is the test most usually employed.

Severe ichthyoses

Rarer and even more severe types of ichthyosis include some in which there is generalized redness (and maybe blistering) as well as generalized scaling. It is important that the affected children are seen and investigated by specialists as there are now treatments for some of these conditions. These children are severely disabled emotionally and socially as well as physically and this should be kept in mind in their management. Also, parents with children suffering from these severe inherited ichthyotic skin disorders should have formal genetic counselling as the inheritance varies according to the particular disorder.

EPIDERMOLYSIS BULLOSA

A further group of congenital skin diseases for which the opinions of a medical geneticist should be obtained is characterized by blistering. The condition is known as epidermolysis bullosa. Some forms are simple and do not cause many problems but others are very severe and cause scarring which results in hideous deformities and is sometimes fatal. Blisters form under the epidermis in response to trauma, and are most frequent on the hands and feet but may occur anywhere, including the mouth.

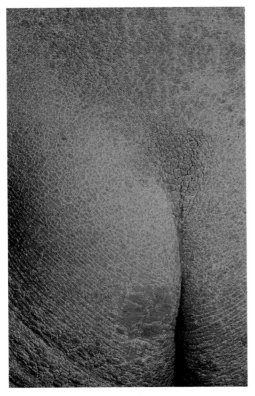

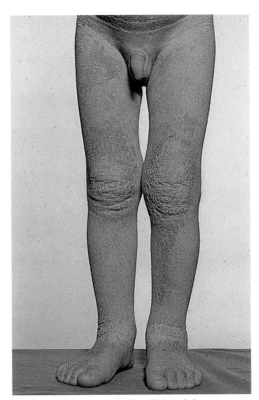

Bullous ichthyosis erythroderma, sometimes known as epidermolytic hyperkeratosis. This is a rare disorder of keratinization, with severe scaling of the skin as well as some redness. In addition, blistering takes place during infancy.

The legs of the same child as below left.

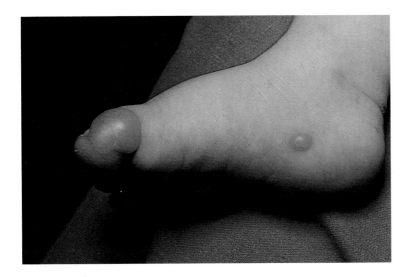

Epidermolysis bullosa. Large tense blisters occur on sites prone to trauma. This child is affected by epidermolysis bullosa simplex, inherited as a dominant trait.

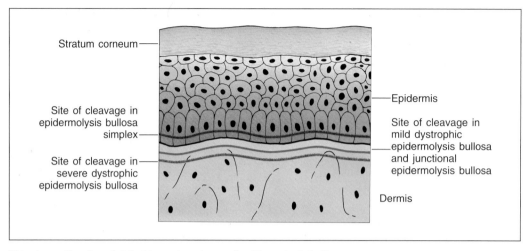

Stratum corneum

Site of cleavage in
epidermolysis bullosa
simplex

Site of cleavage in
severe dystrophic
epidermolysis bullosa

Epidermis

Site of cleavage in
mild dystrophic
epidermolysis bullosa
and junctional
epidermolysis bullosa

Dermis

This shows the sites of defect in various types of epidermolysis bullosa.

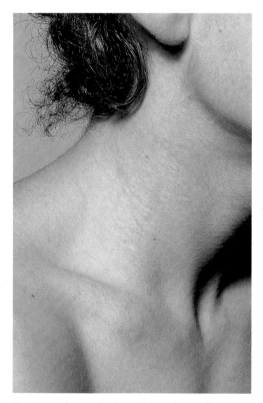

Pseudoxanthoma elasticum. Note the small
yellowish papules along the side of the neck due
to abnormal connective tissue in the dermis. The
condition may affect the connective tissue of many
structures including the cardiovascular system.

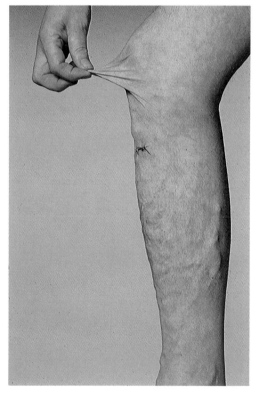

Ehlers Danlos syndrome. The skin is abnormally
hyperelastic. This leads to poor healing of the skin
and formation of broad scars after injury.

If the blisters appear shortly after birth it is very difficult to predict the outcome of the mode of inheritance from the clinical appearance. However, examination of the skin by electron microscope and identification of the exact site of the defect in the skin does give the required information.

OTHER DISORDERS

There are also connective tissue abnormalities that are inherited, including pseudoxanthoma elasticum and the Ehlers Danlos syndrome. These are quite uncommon and the inheritance is complex as the conditions have variants which are inherited differently. These are generalized disorders and, although the condition may present in the skin as fragility of the skin or abnormal scar formation, there are often detectable abnormalities elsewhere in the body as well.

Parents sometimes ask if moles or vascular birthmarks are inherited. In general it is safe to say that they are not, although some rare sorts seem to be.

PRACTICAL POINTS

Some inherited skin diseases
- Most forms of ichthyosis
- Epidermolysis bullosa
- Pseudoxanthoma elasticum
- Ehlers Danlos syndrome

Diseases with a strong genetic element
- Psoriasis
- Atopic dermatitis

5

Skin disease and work

BACKGROUND

It is not generally realized just how disabling skin disease can be. An apparently trivial rash to the observer may be a source of intense discomfort to the sufferer and may make work a nightmare. The physician must take several factors into consideration. First among these is the nature of the disability. A solitary plaque of psoriasis on the trunk is unlikely to cause much in the way of symptoms or any serious functional problem for most occupations. However, I have known a belly dancer with a 2 cm diameter patch of psoriasis around her navel who found that this interfered with her work! This exemplifies the second major consideration, which is the nature of the work of the patient. The average bus driver or postman will not be very concerned by a few warts on the fingers but it may make typing impossible for a secretary. Other factors that have to be taken into account include the economic climate and particular social circumstances of the individual concerned.

DERMATITIS (ECZEMA)

Dermatitis and eczema are synonyms. It is important to understand this because the word 'dermatitis' has developed a special (and unwarranted) significance in everyday language. It has come to mean any rash that is occupationally induced. For this reason, if for no other, the term should only be used with care to patients.

Dermatitis is not a single disease – it is a group of disorders that all show a particular type of epidermal reaction. This may be precipitated by chemical or physical injury, by a specific hypersensitivity to something in the environment or by a constitutional predisposition (atopic dermatitis, for example). Because the reaction is similar regardless of the cause, rashes due to widely differing stimuli may look the same. For this reason it is not easy to determine whether a particular patient's dermatitis rash is due to his occupation or not. It is vital to take a detailed history concerning all potential irritants – both at home and at work – and to keep accurate records for medicolegal purposes. Patch tests to determine whether there are any hypersensitivities will also be required (see Chapter 38). Clearly, when there is any question as to whether the rash has been caused by the patient's work or not, specialist advice should be sought.

The dilemma as to whether to continue work or not is probably most frequently caused by the sudden onset of dermatitis of the hands and/or fingers. To illustrate the key

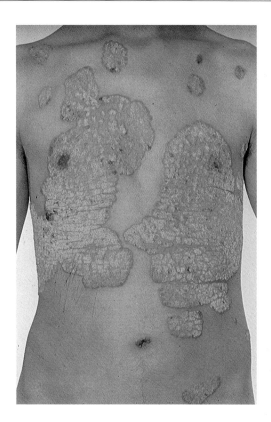

Large plaques of psoriasis which would make it hard for a manual worker to do his job. The lesions are typical, showing a distinct edge and a silvery scale. They started off as small lesions, giving rise to large affected areas.

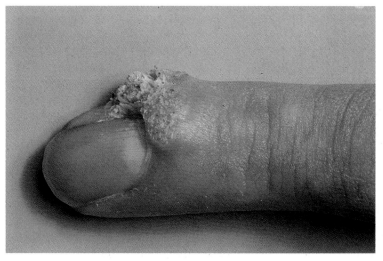

A typical wart on the index finger. This type of paronychial wart can be very difficult to treat. It would not hinder most people from doing their job, but may prevent a typist from working.

Main types of eczema/dermatitis

Type	Name	Synonym	Main clinical manifestations
Endogenous (constitutional)	Atopic	Infantile	Very itchy disorder mainly of flexures and face. Mainly infants.
	Seborrhoeic	—	Scaling areas in scalp and in grooves on face and major body flexures.
	Discoid	Nummular	Disc-shaped scaling areas of limbs.
	Pompholyx	—	Itchy vesicles on palms and soles.
	Lichen simplex chronicus	Circumscribed neurodermatitis	Itchy thickened patch or patches.
Exogenous	Contact allergic	—	At points of contact with sensitizing material but can spread outside. Often acute.
	Contact irritant	'Housewives' dermatitis'	Hands mainly, but may occur on other sites.
	Gravitational	Venous, stasis	Around ankles and lower legs – pigmentation also present.
	Asteatotic	Eczema cracquelée	Legs of elderly mainly affected. Scaling is prominent.
	Light-induced	Photosensitivity dermatitis	In light-exposed areas – often provoked by drugs.

points of diagnosis and management, I will describe four typical, but different, examples of the kind of problems that practitioners can expect to encounter regularly.

Cheiropompholyx

A 19-year-old fireman developed itchy blisters, redness and swelling along the sides of his fingers and on the palms in the ten days before presenting to his doctor. He had never had any previous skin problem and was otherwise fit.

This pattern of dermatitis is sometimes known by the pretentious and confusing name of cheiropompholyx. It is quite often accompanied by the same type of vesicles occurring on the soles of the feet and around the toes. The cause is unknown but is considered to be constitutional in origin although it can be precipitated or aggravated by any stress, physical or emotional.

The patient was very keen to return to work and did not believe that his work was to blame. He was treated at home with wet dressings and weak corticosteroids for one week and given clean, dry work for another two weeks. He was then encouraged to return to

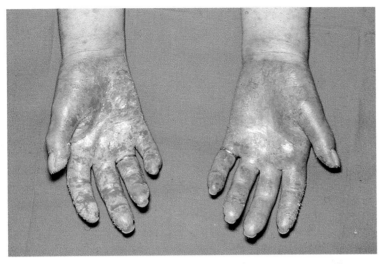

Severe, acute, symmetrical hand dermatitis. The lesions began as small vesicles which wept; the area then became much more inflamed and swollen.

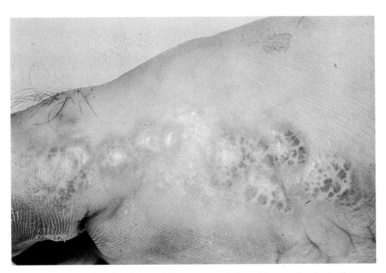

This shows typical coalescing vesicles of pompholyx affecting the foot. The hands and feet are frequently affected together in this type of dermatitic disease.

his normal duties after advice on care of the skin and avoidance of unnecessary injury. He remained well apart from one other episode just before he got married.

'Wear and tear' dermatitis

A 23-year-old mother of two noticed irritant rough scaling and sore cracked patches over the backs and sides of her fingers and on the palms. These had started three months

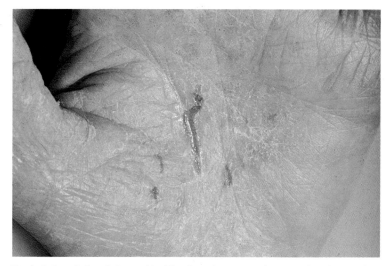

Typical chronic hand dermatitis. The fissuring occurs because the abnormal stratum corneum cracks when the hand extends. This can be very painful and disabling. This was due to persistent physical and mechanical trauma.

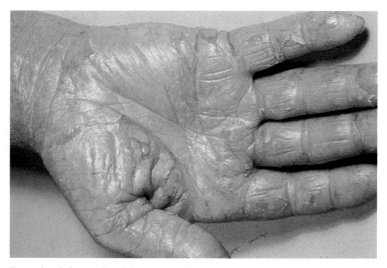

Example of chronic hand dermatitis, due to wear and tear in a motor mechanic.

previously in midwinter and had gradually worsened. Enquiry revealed that she had a part-time job as a domestic cleaner and received little help in the house from her husband.

The picture described was typical of what has come to be known as 'housewives' dermatitis'. It is better described as 'wear and tear' dermatitis as it is the result of persistent or repeated physical and chemical injury to the skin of the hands.

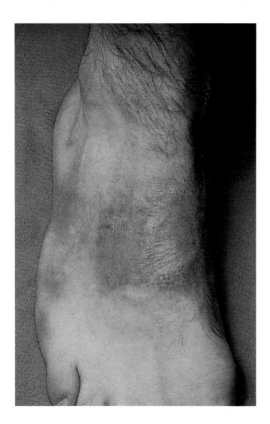

Allergic contact dermatitis on the dorsum of the foot due to sensitivity to a component of a protective shoe worn at work.

She was urged to wear household gloves (cotton gloves under rubber or PVC gloves) while doing housework, to use a simple moisturizing cream, to ask her husband to help out at home as much as possible, and to take a rest from her part-time job. She did not follow this advice and developed an unpleasant infection in one of the cracks that developed on her palms. This solved the problem temporarily as she was admitted to hospital where, away from the traumas of everyday life, her hands healed quickly.

Some occupations at risk from 'wear and tear' dermatitis

- Housewives
- Hairdressers
- Cleaners
- Cooks
- Barmaids
- Mechanics and machinists
- Carpenters
- Nurses
- Builders' labourers
- Miners

Allergic contact dermatitis

A 35-year-old electronics technician developed an irritant red rash that occasionally blistered and wept on the fingers of the hands. When he was first examined it was noticed that the eruption was worse on the right hand and maximal at the tips of the thumb and index fingers. This man remarked that the rash improved at weekends and was almost clear on holidays. It was gradually worsening and beginning to spread up his arms and onto his face and neck. The distribution and nature of the rash and the occupational history was suggestive of an allergic contact dermatitis to one of the materials encountered at work. Patch testing at a later date did in fact reveal a strong positive to epoxy resin – the base material of the glues he was handling every day in the course of his work.

Specialist advice This is urgently required for this type of problem for two reasons. First, a definitive diagnosis is only possible after formal patch testing by someone with experience (see Chapters 34 and 38). Second, expert advice is necessary concerning what to avoid in future and what can be handled with impunity. It is not uncommon for such patients to resort to litigation (this one, in fact, did), and it is better to have an informed opinion early on in the march of events rather than later when all symptoms have abated and the history is hazy.

Treatment When there is a strong suspicion that occupational exposure is the cause of a rapidly worsening eruption, as in this case, it is foolhardy to permit the individual to return to work until the condition has completely subsided.

The acute stage, when the rash is swollen, sore and blistering, should be treated by saline compresses or bathing in dilute potassium permanganate solution (1:8000). A little later, bland emollient creams are useful. If no further exposure occurs the rash will often settle within three or four weeks, but it is quite common for it to flare up unexpectedly. Whether this is due to unmentioned or unknown exposure to the allergen, or whether this happens independently of further contact with the sensitizing agent, is not known.

Return to work After a few weeks the patient and the physician are often both bored with the problem. At this stage it is quite tempting to suggest a return to work. If arrangements can be made for the patient to do only clean, dry, non-manual work, well away from the sensitizer, then this may be the best plan. But make no mistake, even this sometimes provokes a fresh crop of spots.

Some occupations at risk from allergic contact dermatitis

- Photographers
- Nurses
- Dental technicians
- Chemical workers
- Horticulturists
- Rubber industry workers
- Electroplating workers

There was no choice for the electronics technician but to try to change jobs. As far as the company was concerned he was no use to them unless he could handle the adhesive containing the epoxy resin, and anyway the atmosphere had been soured by the legal process resulting from the claim he had made. In times such as these, when employment is at a premium, such decisions are difficult, but this man's best option was to agree with the employers and try to find work elsewhere, well away from epoxy resin glues.

Atopic dermatitis

The last example concerns a 19-year-old nurse in her second year of training. She was referred to me by the occupational health service of the hospital, who said that she had developed 'an itchy skin problem' affecting the hands, arms, face and scattered patches elsewhere. It turned out that her father was asthmatic and that she suffered from hay fever and had always had an itchy dry skin and a few scaling itchy patches. Clearly she was suffering from a mild type of late-onset atopic dermatitis. Sometimes, as in this patient, the brunt of the disease does fall on the hands and then diagnosis can be quite difficult. Of course, patch tests were carried out just to be certain that she did not in fact have some type of allergic contact dermatitis to one of the drugs she often handled (such as penicillin). All patch tests were negative. She was a bright

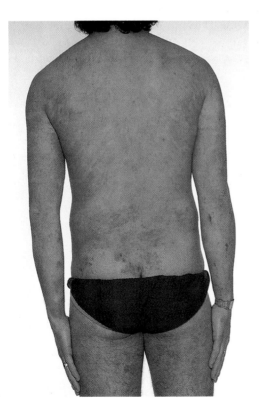

Generalized atopic dermatitis. This patient was quite distressed by his persistently itching dermatitic rash. Scratch marks can be seen around the elbows and buttocks. This eruption would make it impossible to work in a hot, sweaty environment, such as on a hot factory floor.

and keen young woman who was alarmed at the thought of being kept off work by a rash.

Return to work This type of problem can be quite difficult and there is no easy formula to apply. Each patient should be carefully evaluated to assess:

1. Their keenness for their present job.
2. The disability caused by the skin problem.
3. The role of the job in causing, precipitating or aggravating the rash.
4. The potential danger to workmates or the public by continuing to work with the rash.
5. The attitudes of the employers.

The nurse was keen and popular with patients and the nursing hierarchy. Although the job had obviously precipitated and then aggravated her constitutional dermatitis she could be given jobs that were less damaging to the skin than routine nursing duties. However, it had to be arranged that she did not assist at sterile procedures or dress wounds, because damaged, scaling skin can easily be colonized by pathogenic bacteria. Good nursing recruits were particularly difficult to find in the area. For all these reasons it was decided that she should continue her nursing studies. I am not sorry now that we made this decision, as she is now an excellent senior nurse involved in teaching!

PSORIASIS

Psoriasis is a common, persistent or recurrent inflammatory skin disorder in adults, whose cause is unknown. It seems that there is a strong genetic element, although this is not evident in every case. The large majority of sufferers go through life with a few psoriatic plaques or have just one attack with more generalized lesions (see Chapter 19). For these comparatively lucky people the disease is no bar to work of any type. Unfortunately there are several groups of psoriatics whose skin problem interferes with their work.

Psoriasis of the hands and/or feet

Ordinary scaly psoriasis and a form of pustular psoriasis can affect the hands and the feet. It is usually the palms and soles that are involved. Although these may be the only sites affected, the resultant disability can be quite out of proportion to the extent of the disease. The horny layer of the palms and soles needs to be tough yet elastic for proper function. When it is abnormal, as in psoriasis, it tends to crack. The cracks that form can become inflamed and very painful, just as in dermatitis. This discomfort can prevent ordinary use of the hands and may even make walking difficult.

Psoriasis tends to appear at the sites of injury. This is known as the isomorphic response (the Koebner phenomenon). For this reason attacks of psoriasis can be precipitated by tough manual work. Similarly, patches of psoriasis can be made worse if subjected to perpetual minor irritation. Patients differ in the way that they react to injury, and so advice has to be tailored to the individual.

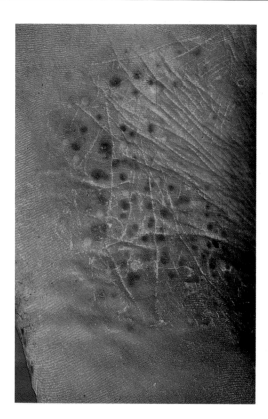

Pustular psoriasis (sometimes called pustulosis) affecting the sole. There are many new yellowish pustules and many dark red or brown older lesions. Eventually the area becomes cracked and scaling, making any job that involves a great deal of walking or standing extremely difficult.

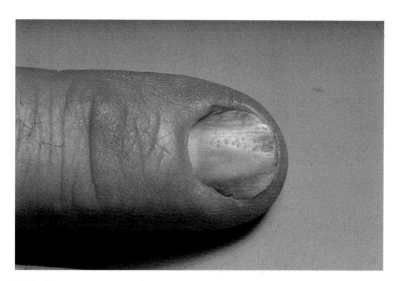

Nail pitting in psoriasis is fairly common. This example also shows the feature of onycholysis and some nail-plate abnormality, both of which are also quite common in this disease.

If the nails are particularly badly involved other problems can arise. The pitting and discolouration are unsightly but it is the separation of nail plate from nail bed (onycholysis) that causes most complaints and can make some jobs very difficult. Needlework or work requiring delicate manipulations such as in the electronics industry are two such examples. Office work, particularly typing, can also be a trial if there is extensive involvement of the fingernails.

When psoriasis affects the hands there is also the problem of the general public's reaction to its appearance. I have known several waiters who virtually have had to look for other types of work because their employers have said that they could not serve at table while their hands were affected.

It must also be remembered that ointment or cream treatments become difficult for those who work with their hands. Most topical applications are in some degree greasy and will tend to rub off and soil paper or other materials that need to be handled.

Psoriasis of the body and limbs

Unless there are many large patches of psoriasis it is not usual for the chronic plaque type of psoriasis on the body or limbs to interfere much with work. The individual patches are sometimes sore but apart from the occasional cosmetic difficulty they should not cause problems with an occupation. When it affects the flexures, as it does

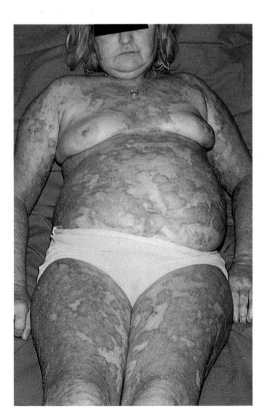

Typical widespread psoriasis. There is involvement of between 65 and 70 per cent of the body area in this patient, and she felt cold because of the loss of heat from the skin surface. Psoriasis of this severity makes it very hard to do any kind of work at all.

occasionally, it can cause considerable soreness and discomfort, and then does interfere with mobility.

Sweating is defective in plaques of psoriasis, probably because the sweat ducts are blocked by abnormal horn. This can make life difficult for those with widespread disease who work in the heat – boilermen, for example. If you can't sweat you can't lose heat, and hyperpyrexia may result.

In erupting, active psoriasis affecting 30 per cent or more of this skin surface there is another problem. The increased blood flow causes heat loss, and in the severest cases can result in hypothermia. Obviously, outdoor work in the cold is not advisable for psoriatics in an eruptive phase.

There have been reports of bacterial colonization of the chronically scaling lesions of plaque-type psoriasis and the infection of surgical wounds by psoriatic medical staff. Nurses, surgeons and other operating theatre staff of all types should have regular bacterial swabs and preferably should avoid direct contact with open wounds while their psoriasis is active.

Unjustified bar to employment In some occupations in which there is a pre-employment medical examination the discovery of psoriasis is a bar to being accepted. I find this illogical. The one predictable thing about psoriasis is its unpredictability. There is no way of knowing whether someone with a small patch of psoriasis will remain someone with a small patch of psoriasis, become totally disabled by universal psoriasis or become rash-free and rise to be another Henry Ford! Although there are no statistics to prove it, experience tells me that excessive loss of time from work because of psoriasis is the exception rather than the rule. In my view, exclusion from a particular job because of psoriasis should only occur after considerable heart-searching and after consideration of the work involved as well as the individual's ability to do it, at the time of examination.

ACNE

It is more common than generally thought for acne to cause an occupational problem. Severe acne with deep cystic lesions may be very painful and the lesions are sometimes so tender that it becomes impossible to wear a collar or anything on the shoulders. Luckily such severe episodes usually respond to treatment (see Chapter 21) and are short-lived. A few unfortunates are persistently severely affected and it can be difficult for them to tackle a heavy labouring job or continue work in a uniformed service.

Acne can suddenly become explosively severe in moist tropical climates, especially when there are few opportunities for frequent bathing and rest in air-conditioned surroundings. This type of so-called 'tropical acne' was the cause of a great deal of evacuation from Far-Eastern war zones in recent conflicts there. The possibility of acne behaving in this way in young men who are likely to serve abroad under such circumstances should be remembered during pre-employment examinations.

Problems of appearance

It is more usual for acne to cause employment problems in another way. The prejudice that the media have created in favour of the ideal body image can result in difficulties for the youngster with bad facial acne – especially in jobs which involve meeting

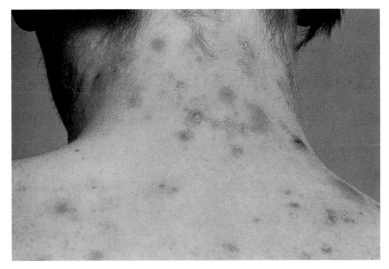

This young man's severe acne proved disabling for him as it affected the back of the neck and rubbed against his collar.

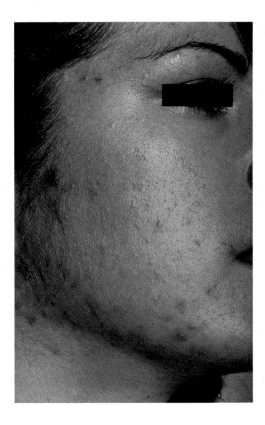

Mild acne is extremely common. This shows a young woman with typical papules and comedones.

Some occupations made difficult by severe acne

● Bakers
● Boilermakers
● Soldiers and other uniformed services
● Actors

the public. This situation is exemplified by the case of a 23-year-old saleswoman with recurrent attacks of large papules and nodules on the forehead, cheeks and chin who worked in a small but smart clothes boutique. The manageress was concerned (unduly in my opinion) that customers would not want to be served by her, and so she was either told to go home while her acne was bad or made to do some menial job in the stockroom.

Another way in which acne can interfere with work may actually be more common and concerns the affected person's own conception of the way he or she looks. An 18-year-old girl desperately wanted to be a hairdresser but because of relatively minor acne blemishes decided to work in a factory. She felt that the clients would be horrified at her appearance. Firm reassurance is required for this sort of patient, though I am sad to say it rarely seems effective.

Acne can always be improved by treatment with topical agents such as tretinoin or isotretinoin preparations or benzoyl-peroxide-containing gel (Panoxyl) or systemic antibiotics (see Chapter 21) and, in the large majority of cases, subsides spontaneously after two or three years. During the time it is present sympathy and understanding are required for the problems that sometimes arise.

Occupational acne

The other side of the coin is occupational acne or acne aggravated by work. Tropical acne, mentioned previously, can be considered occupational in some cases. It is sometimes said that ordinary acne may be aggravated by hot and sweaty jobs such as baking or stoking, and it must be admitted that acne among those working in these professions does seem to improve after a spell away from work.

Frequent contact of hair-bearing skin with lubricating and cutting oils and greases can produce a type of acne. This may occur over the front of the thighs from oil-soaked overalls, and on the forearms. Although unpleasant it clears fairly quickly once contact with the oils responsible is prevented.

A more serious type of acne is that associated with exposure to small amounts of the chemical agent known as dioxin and chlorphenols used extensively in industry for insulation. There have been several incidents at chemical plants in recent years in which explosions or other accidents have resulted in contamination of the surrounding environment with chemicals of this sort, and subsequently in cases of 'chloracne'. Chloracne can be very unpleasant and persistent with many large and painful cysts.

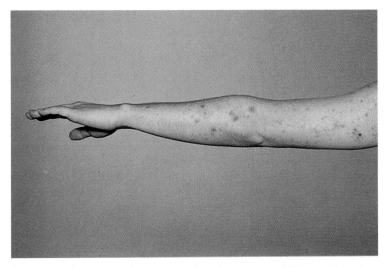

Acne of the shoulders and upper arms is not uncommon. When it affects the forearms, as in this patient, an occupational cause is likely. His job as a machine minder was dirty and his clothes became oil soaked, causing acne in several unusual areas.

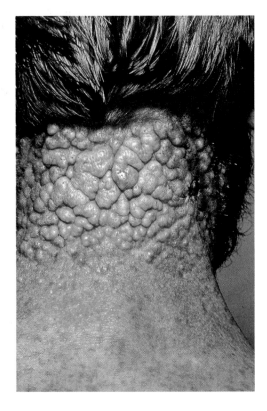

The back of the neck of a middle-aged chemical plant worker who developed dreadful cystic acne.

OTHER SKIN DISEASES

Clearly it is not possible in a book of this size to explore all the complex interactions between skin disease and work. So far I have tried to describe the most common problems that arise in this context. Other types of difficulty may arise from skin disorders caused by infectious agents. It is especially important here that each individual case be judged on its own merits. A secretary can continue to work with herpes simplex cold sores around the lips but nurses and doctors who may come into contact with patients who are vulnerable to infection should not. Food handlers should be excluded from work if they have any type of infected skin lesion until there are no further signs of infection, but there are few dangers in permitting someone to continue work on a car assembly line if they are able to do so.

PRACTICAL POINTS

- The importance to patients of successful treatment of a skin disease is often that it enables them to return to work.
- The decision to keep a patient with a skin disorder away from work has to be based on the particular circumstances of each individual.
- When dermatitis is diagnosed as due to a substance or substances in the working environment, the patient should be advised to take every precaution to avoid contact with the allergen or, if this is not possible, to change jobs.
- It is important to watch for problems of heat intolerance and heat loss in patients with widespread psoriasis or other generalized rashes.
- Firm reassurance combined with vigorous treatment is required for young acne patients whose facial appearance is creating problems at work.

6
Skin disease and vacations

BACKGROUND

Literally millions of citizens living in Europe pack up and go on vacation for 2–4 weeks each year. Holiday entitlement has greatly increased since 1945 and leisure activities are now an important aspect of the 'life plan' of an individual. People in countries outside Europe may not have so long for vacations at the moment but the tendency is for everyone to want to spend time outside of their usual environment. In this short chapter I will discuss two types of problem associated with vacations – the effect of vacation on pre-existing skin disease, and skin disorders that may result from being on holiday.

EFFECTS OF PRE-EXISTING SKIN DISEASE

Psoriasis

Most patients with ordinary plaque-type psoriasis cope very well with going on vacation – as long as they remember to take their medication with them! In fact many improve because of the rest and increased sun exposure. Those with extensive psoriasis have special problems because of the large amount of scale that is shed and because of difficulties that may be experienced with special bathing requirements and the need for dressings.

Atopic dermatitis

Much the same can be said about patients with atopic dermatitis as with patients with psoriasis. There are a few special points that should be noted for this group – the ease with which they develop skin infections and their skin becomes irritated may cause problems. While some patients with atopic dermatitis really benefit by judicious sun exposure others cannot tolerate the sun or the heat and may worsen. Another problem is the persistent pruritus and the bleeding excoriations that severely affected atopics may have. The bedclothes and towels may become soiled – adding to the patient's unpopularity.

Acne

The only potential problem for patients with acne arises if they are in a hot humid climate and are unable to 'cool off' and bathe or shower as usual. Their acne may become dramatically worse.

SKIN DISEASE RESULTING FROM VACATION

What could be healthier than taking a rest in pleasant and different surroundings? Yet holidaymakers develop odd rashes because, as most physicians in holiday resort towns will tell you, people on vacation submit themselves quite willingly to quite silly extremes and are seemingly oblivious to obvious health hazards.

Problems from sun exposure

We differ in our sensitivity to the sun's ultraviolet rays according to our degree of skin pigmentation and individual susceptibility. Few take heed of the warnings not to spend too much time in the midday sun, or listen to the advice concerning sunscreens (see pages 59–60). Severe sunburn is unfortunately only too common. Affected individuals are often in acute agony for a few days and may feel quite unwell. Most will not need treatment other than a soothing emollient cream, but more severely affected patients may require topical corticosteroids. Aspirin may help the skin inflammation in some cases.

Uncommonly, sun exposure may precipitate one of the photodermatoses such as porphyria cutanea tarda or 'polymorphic light eruption'. Sun exposure can also precipitate a photosensitivity – a number of drugs taken systemically or used topically can cause a 'photodermatitis' (see pages 92–95).

The sun may reactivate herpes simplex or precipitate erythema multiforme. The sun's heat may also be the cause of skin problems because of the increased amount of sweating. If the skin does not have the chance to cool and dry off, the surface becomes macerated and the sweat pores become blocked. This causes 'sweat rash' (or miliaria). If quite superficial a tiny clear vesicle is produced. If the blockage is deeper down an inflamed papule is produced. These lesions often occur on the neck and around the flexures.

Other environmental hazards

Unfortunately, the most exotic and alluring of holiday destinations aren't always the most 'skin-friendly'. The nuisance of minor bites and stings from flying and crawling insects (see Chapter 14) is enough to make some wish they were back in the relative safety of their offices!

Plant life can also be disappointingly aggressive. Contact with 'poison ivy' in North America can cause dreadful eczema at the sites of contact, as can poison oak in Europe (but less frequently). Some plants, such as giant hogweed, are photosensitizers and can cause an unpleasant photodermatitis.

PRACTICAL POINTS

- Patients with severe generalized psoriasis or atopic dermatitis need to plan their holidays with care and continue with medication while away.
- A major problem for those on vacation can be excessive sun exposure resulting in severe sunburn or a photodermatosis. Adequate sunscreens should be used to prevent such problems.
- Other unaccustomed environmental challenges including insect bites and stings and contact with certain plants may also cause skin problems.

7

Skin problems in the elderly

BACKGROUND

The ever-increasing number of citizens over the age of 60 means that the elderly will constitute an increasingly important aspect of medical practice for the foreseeable future. This is particularly true for dermatology as health problems of the skin figure disproportionately in the process of growing old. Most of the common skin diseases (dermatitis, psoriasis, lichen planus) affect the skin of the elderly in the same way as they do in other age groups. However, flexural psoriasis is more frequently found in older age groups; curiously, atopic dermatitis is also not uncommon.

With increasing age two processes relentlessly progress to impair the appearance and function of the skin. The first and most important is the cumulated environmental injury, resulting in most cases from climatic damage to the skin of different kinds, and possibly also from long-term exposure to detergent substances or solvents and minor mechanical trauma – such as from ill-fitting shoes or repeated abrasion. The second is the poorly understood but inevitable series of changes that occur as a result of true biological ageing.

CLIMATIC INJURY DUE TO SUN EXPOSURE

Most climatic skin problems are caused by exposure to the sun; the outdoor life may do wonders for the morale but it gradually destroys the skin. Sailors, farmers, fishermen, builders and sportsmen are among the occupational groups that are particularly at risk. The damaging effect of the sun is also a problem for obsessional sunbathers and others who spend most of their leisure time out of doors in sunny weather. The lighter the complexion, the more vulnerable is the skin to this type of injury. People with Celtic ancestry are especially at risk. The degree of solar damage is dependent on the cumulative dose received and the dose is proportional to both the intensity of the sun and the length of time spent in it. Clearly, 30 minutes spent on an Australian beach may be equivalent to three or four hours in an English seaside resort during an average British summer! It is the invisible ultraviolet part of the sun's spectrum that causes the damage and in general the hotter and brighter the sun, the more ultraviolet light there is.

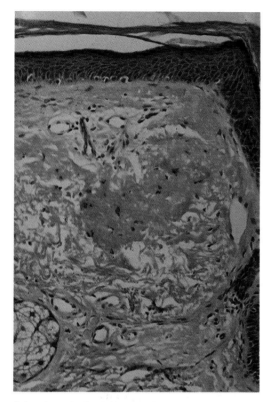

Solar elastotic degeneration of connective tissue (solar elastosis). The connective tissue in the upper dermis is disorganized without the usual fibrillar pattern, and has different staining properties from normal connective tissue.

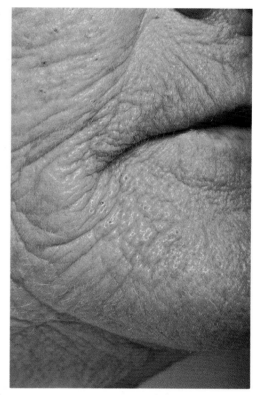

This type of wrinkling is often mistakenly thought to be due to age. It is in fact due to chronic solar damage causing elastotic degenerative change in the upper dermis.

Other effects of chronic sun exposure

A major effect of chronic sun exposure is a particular change in the upper dermal connective tissue. The tissue loses its usual fibrillar appearance, becomes disorganized and takes on the staining appearance of elastic tissue. Paradoxically, the elastotic dermis loses the normal elastic properties of connective tissue and this causes the wrinkling and sagging seen in the skin of the elderly. The same changes also occur in the not so elderly who have spent their early years as sun worshippers. There is clearly an individual susceptibility to the development of this change which is not entirely dependent on the degree of skin pigmentation. However, not all the reasons for a particular individual's sensitivity to the sun are known.

Apart from the wrinkled appearances which most regard as ugly and undesirable, such damaged skin is prone to other types of blemish. Crimson bruises known as senile purpura, which take many weeks to disappear, develop over the forearms. The backs of the hands and the sides of the face develop flat brown lesions called 'senile

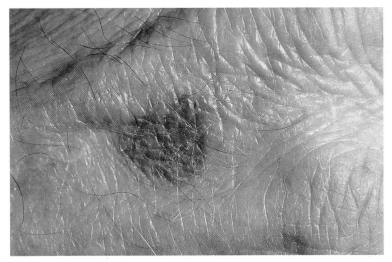

Senile purpura. These purplish patches appear on the arms mainly in the elderly who have elastotic degeneration of the connective tissue. They do not have any haematological significance.

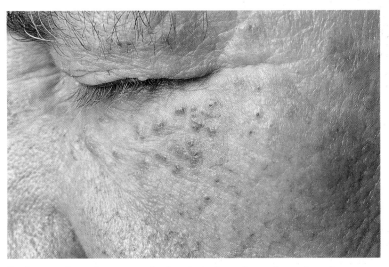

Senile comedones in an area of solar elastosis on the malar region of a woman in late middle age.

lentigines'. On the upper cheeks large blackheads may appear, known appropriately as senile comedones. The relationship of these lesions to solar damage is uncertain. Curious angular or stellate scar-like lesions sometimes develop on the backs of hands or forearms. These changes do not cause much in the way of symptoms, but may cause considerable psychological discomfiture on account of their appearance.

Effects of chronic sun exposure

- Wrinkling and sagging skin
- Senile purpura
- Senile lentigines and comedones
- Angular and stellate scar-like lesions
- Solar keratoses
- Bowen's disease and squamous cell carcinoma
- Basal cell carcinoma
- Malignant melanoma

Treatments

Women in particular may be very disturbed by the appearance of wrinkles and blemishes and, if they are wealthy enough, may try anything and everything to rid themselves of the unwanted signs of solar damage. 'Antiwrinkle creams' may marginally improve appearance transiently, but do less than their manufacturers claim and cost the earth. It is claimed that various superficial acid peeling treatments help, but these may cause more discomfort than improvement. Glycolic acid (65–70 per cent), one of the alpha-hydroxy acids or so-called 'fruit acids', has been much used for this purpose in the past few years and has been claimed to give excellent cosmetic results. Facelifts by skilled cosmetic surgeons can cunningly disguise some facial wrinkling and neck bagginess. It is now established that topical tretinoin (and isotretinoin) when

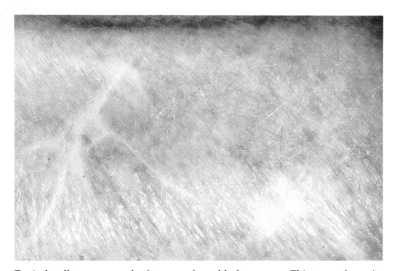

Typical stellate scars on the forearm of an elderly woman. This type of scar is due to elastotic degeneration of dermal connective tissue. It is often rationalized by its owner as being due to trauma but is mainly due to the effects of solar damage.

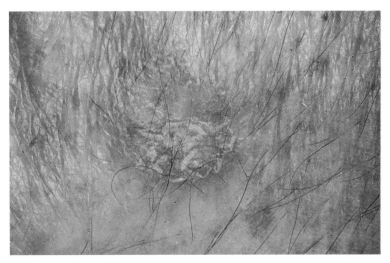

Senile keratosis on the back of an elderly woman's hand. These lesions are usually red and have an adherent scale.

used daily on the affected areas will, over a period of months, gradually decrease the fine lines, sallow appearance and senile lentigines due to photoageing. This improvement in photodamaged skin also occurs with topical isotretinoin. It seems to be due to the topical retinoids stimulating the production of both new epidermal cells and new dermal constituents.

Whatever remedial treatment is undertaken, it is very much a case of shutting the stable door after the horse has bolted. I believe that it is useful to tell patients who complain of these problems to avoid excessive sun exposure from then on, in the hope that this will stop progression of the disorder which may then also spontaneously improve.

GROWTHS CAUSED BY CHRONIC SUN EXPOSURE

Squamous cell cancer

The epidermis develops small warty precancerous lesions known as solar (or senile) keratoses (see also page 78). They occur most frequently on the dorsa of the hands, on the forehead, the nose, the tops of the ears and, in men, on the bald area of the scalp. Most of these small warty excrescences either just enlarge extremely slowly or remain unchanged for many years, or even disappear spontaneously. However, a tiny proportion (perhaps as small as 0.1 per cent) becomes aggressive and develops into frank squamous cell cancers. Rapid enlargement and/or ulceration are signs of this change. The most important point about solar keratoses is not that they have a potential to transform into a squamous cell carcinoma, but that their presence signifies that the skin has sustained significant solar damage. Squamous cell carcinomas are at best locally destructive and, even worse, sometimes metastasize.

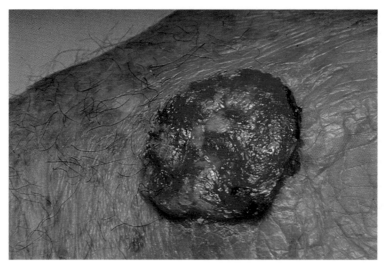

Squamous cell carcinoma on the back of a hand. This developed over the space of a few weeks in an elderly man. Previously there had been a scaling area present, which presumably was a solar keratosis.

Basal cell carcinoma (rodent ulcer)

This is another result of chronic solar damage. It starts as a small dome-shaped pearly nodule which breaks down centrally to give rise to a spreading ulcer with raised margins. These lesions, while slow growing, can eventually become extremely mutilating and always need speedy treatment. While most are the result of sun exposure, some occur in non-exposed sites and clearly have other causes.

Malignant melanoma

This is the most unpleasant skin cancer to result from solar injury. It is true that this neoplasm is not a prerogative of any age group, but it does occur among the elderly and so is worth mentioning here as another (and awful) consequence of persistent sun exposure (see also pages 218–19).

Seborrhoeic warts

These benign pigmented warty lesions appear in middle life and gradually increase in number (see also pages 220–1). They are particularly common in areas exposed to light, but may be seen anywhere and are often particularly prolific over the trunk. They are frequently confused with malignant melanoma because of their dark brown or even black colour, but melanoma is almost never warty. They also need to be distinguished from pigmented basal cell carcinoma, which is also hardly ever warty; and from solar keratosis, which is occasionally slightly pigmented.

Seborrhoeic warts mostly do not need treatment but if it is thought that they need to be removed the best plan is to curette them off using local anaesthesia and to lightly cauterize the base. This should not leave a scar, and they rarely seem to return at the site of removal.

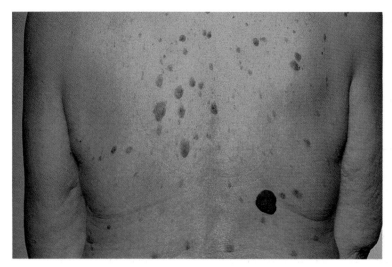

Multiple seborrhoeic warts on the back of a 60-year-old lady. These lesions are usually pigmented and have a slightly greasy, warty surface.

ERYTHEMA AB IGNE

This disorder is seen on the front of the lower legs in elderly folk who sit in front of a coal, gas or electric fire over long periods. There is a net-like pattern of reddish-brown markings due to the infrared radiation received from the focal heat source. Uncommonly squamous cell cancer can arise in such a 'chronically burnt area'.

THE BIOLOGICAL EFFECTS OF AGEING ON THE SKIN

Dry skin

The epidermal cells become smaller and the cells of the stratum corneum produced by the epidermis – the corneocytes – become larger in area. Also, the rate of epidermal cell production is decreased in the elderly. In themselves these changes do not appear to result in a significant abnormality of function. However, it is more than likely that they are partially responsible for the apparent dryness and scaliness of the skin of elderly people. This is associated with a distressing itchiness that is heightened in the winter and in the dry atmosphere of central heating.

Treatment Treatment for itching and dryness of elderly skin is inadequate, as it is for most types of itchiness (see pages 112–13). Emollient soaps and lotions are of some help as is the application of mentholated preparations e.g. 0.5 per cent menthol in oily calamine lotion (see page 112). Too frequent bathing for too long in hot water with vigorous scrubbing and towelling will aggravate the symptoms. Tepid showering and patting dry afterwards is kinder to the skin.

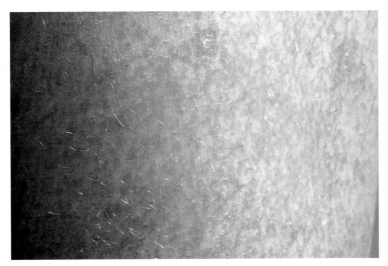

Dry, itchy skin in the elderly can be very distressing for such patients. The skin is roughened and in this patient eczematous change is beginning (eczema craquelée).

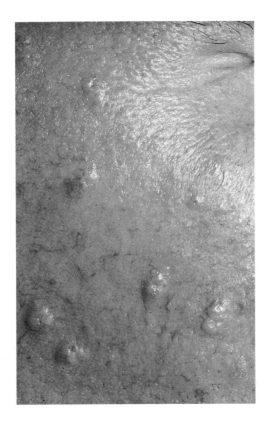

Senile sebaceous gland hypertrophy. The lesions seen in this condition are benign and are often confused with basal cell carcinoma (see page 220).

Changes in sweating and enlargement of sebaceous glands

Sweating tends to be less in old age. The rate of sebum secretion from the oil glands of the hair follicles tends to be maintained at normal adult levels until the seventh decade and then is gradually reduced. Curiously it increases in patients with Parkinsonism. There is a paradoxical enlargement of the sebaceous glands on the face in some elderly individuals; it is not known whether this is due to some curious hormonal change or the result of climatic damage to the surrounding dermal connective tissue.

Impaired wound healing

The dermal connective tissue gradually thins with increasing age, and becomes less elastic and compliant. These changes may partly explain the reduced vigour of wound healing in elderly people. The epidermis is also less able to repair defects in its continuity.

Reduction in immunocompetence

It should also be remembered that there is a reduction in immunocompetence in old age and infective disorders may be devastating to this age group. Erysipelas, while not common now, still occurs and can be a life-threatening disease. Red, swollen, tender, sharply defined areas on the face or legs, accompanied by systemic upset, must be

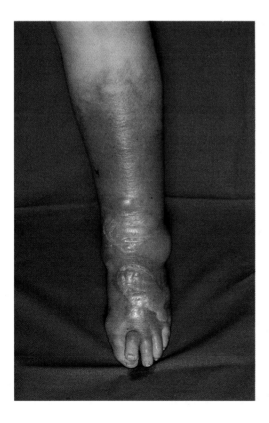

Erysipelas can be a very serious disease. Prior to antibiotics it used to be a killer. The affected area is usually intensely red and may even be purpuric. Blistering sometimes occurs, as here.

urgently treated with antibiotics. Penicillin is the first treatment of choice. If improvement does not occur rapidly, specialist advice should be sought.

The skin of the feet

This is often an area of trouble and the cause of much disability in the elderly. Years of tight-fitting fashionable shoes cause painful deformed feet with calluses, corns and bunions. A chiropodist's advice is invaluable for those afflicted in this way. Flat comfortable shoes, regular paring of the hard skin by the chiropodist or by somebody trained to do this and the use of emollients or salicylic acid preparations (see page 115) will all be helpful.

Deformed toe-nails are also troublesome. Thickened, yellowish and misshapen nails may be the result of ringworm or psoriasis but also seem to occur without any easily identifiable cause in the elderly. They are difficult to cut and keep tidy – largely because of the decreased mobility of the senior citizen – and assistance is often required for this aspect of their routine toilet.

The skin of the legs

Venous hypertension The effects of venous hypertension are a frequent cause of problems of the skin of the lower legs in this age group. Dilated venules coursing over the skin of the ankle and instep do not usually give rise to symptoms, but are frequently accompanied by dusky brown pigmentation from deposits of haemosiderin. The skin eventually becomes taut and loses its normal elasticity due to gradual tissue fibrosis. Gravitational eczema can occur at any stage of this process, causing pruritus and giving rise to ill-characterized aches and discomfort in the legs. Ulceration is also a frequent and unpleasant complication of

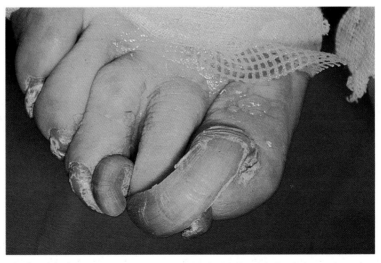

Abnormality of the toe-nails is quite common in the elderly. It can cause needless disability, as regular chiropody should prevent the type of change seen here.

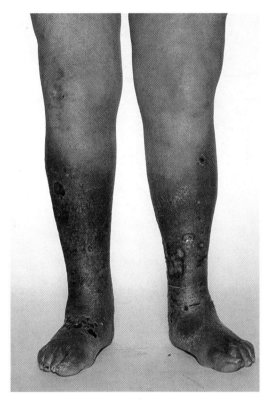 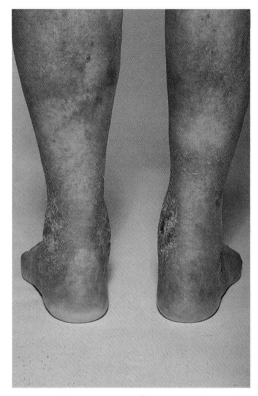

Dusky pigmentation around the ankles and lower legs in the elderly is mostly due to venous incompetence. Small amounts of blood seep into the tissues and are broken down to give rise to staining by haemosiderin.

Gravitational eczema frequently accompanies venous incompetence. Often it is due to an allergy to topical treatments used for the condition. For an unknown reason the skin of the lower legs in these patients is very easily sensitized.

chronic gravitational eczema (see Chapter 23). The ulceration of the ankles or lower legs may become infected and painful. It is always a source of discomfort and disability.

Ischaemic changes These are also a potent source of problems in the skin of the legs in old age. Small necrotic areas appear over the toes, the dorsum of the foot, the heel or the lower leg around the ankles. 'Nutritional' changes also occur in the skin in ischaemia, with loss of hair and a general appearance of atrophy. Ischaemic change is generally painful in contrast to venous ulceration which, although uncomfortable, is uncommonly as painful. Specialist opinion should be sought for its management, as vascular surgery has much to offer some patients.

Dry skin The skin of the legs is also particularly prone to the dry skin problems mentioned earlier in this chapter. Sometimes this may progress to a type of dermatitis known as 'asteatotic eczema' or 'eczema craquelée', where the skin takes on a kind of 'crazy paving' appearance. Dry, scaling and fissured areas appear over the shins and thighs. They may also occur over the upper arms and back but are less often seen

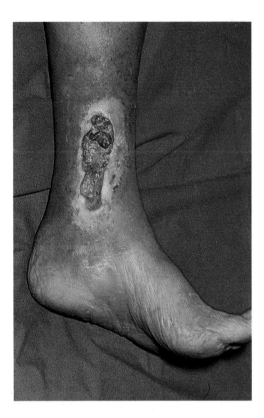

A typical venous ulcer occurring just above the medial malleolus. The base is relatively clean and the edge sodden, indicating that the lesion has been treated recently with airtight dressings. Note that there is pigmentation around the ulcer and that there is also some dusky redness due to subsiding inflammation.

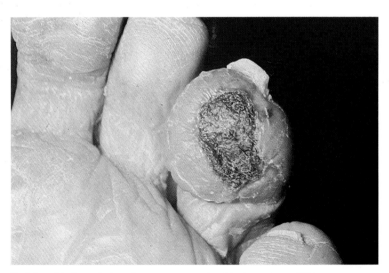

Peripheral ischaemia is only too common in elderly patients. This man complained of painful areas on his feet which were cold to the touch. The photograph shows a bluish area on his middle toe, the tip of which has started to necrose and ulcerate.

elsewhere. This condition responds rapidly to bland emollient preparations and to avoidance of vigorous skin toilet, rather than to corticosteroid preparations.

PROBLEMS OF MANAGEMENT

When prescribing for the elderly, the diminished capacity for compliance with complex instructions should be borne in mind. Not only may the senior citizen be unable to understand the instructions given or be unable to remember them adequately, but he or she may be physically incapable or carrying them out. Reduced mobility and arthritis may prevent the regular application of topical treatments. Social and economic hardship (unfortunately frequent in the older age groups) may prevent regular bathing, adequate diet or adequate clothing. The practitioner should make full use of whatever nursing help and social welfare agencies are available to ensure that the necessary treatments are given at the correct time.

PRACTICAL POINTS

- The appearances of ageing in the elderly are due either to previous chronic sun exposure or to the biological effects of ageing.
- Wrinkling, senile lentigines and other effects due to chronic photodamage may be improved by emollients, sun protection and the use of topical retinoids.
- Practitioners should be alert to the possibility of squamous cell cancer, basal cell carcinoma and malignant melanoma on sundamaged skin in the elderly. Distinguish carefully between seborrhoeic warts and malignant melanoma.
- The itchiness commonly associated with dry skin in the elderly can be alleviated with emollient soaps and lotions. Tepid showers followed by gentle patting dry should be recommended to replace the more usual routine of baths and vigorous towelling.
- Disorders in the skin of the legs are particularly common in the older age group and include:
  –Gravitational eczema
  –Gravitational ulcers
  –Painful necrotic areas in the lower legs and feet caused by ischaemic changes
  –Asteatotic eczema
  –Erythema ab igne (due to persistent exposure to focal heating).

8

Psyche and skin disease

BACKGROUND

The idea that skin disease is caused by 'nerves' has deep roots in the popular imagination. What is more, the 'roots' are frequently watered by many of my well-meaning practitioner colleagues. There is no firm evidence of which I am aware that suggests that common skin disorders are caused by stress, anxiety or depression. All human ailments (including cancer and the trauma of road accidents) may be precipitated by stress, and of course we all know that stress may aggravate some disease. But there is a world of difference between this type of relationship and a causative role. These remarks apply to such common disorders as psoriasis, atopic dermatitis, rosacea and urticaria.

It is common to hear from patients that their rash flares up just before an exam or at a time of marital strife; atopic dermatitis is notoriously unstable in this respect. Rosacea is also subject to relapses after a stressful experience.

NEUROSIS-RELATED CONDITIONS

In some less common skin disorders there is a closer link between the mind and the skin. For example, on rare occasions skin lesions are purposely caused by people who are conventionally dubbed 'hysterical'. Ulcers, dermatitic rashes and bizarre inflammatory lesions may be physically produced by these patients. Recognition of the artefactual nature of a skin disease can sometimes be very difficult, requiring the acumen and understanding of a dermatological Hercule Poirot.

There are also some disorders in which one suspects that the initial skin problem was trivial but that anxiety or some other neurotic reaction has magnified it or has been responsible for its persistence. I am thinking in particular of patients with pruritus ani or pruritus vulvae (see Chapter 17). Some of these unfortunates have had their symptoms for many years and have been unsuccessfully investigated in turn by practitioner, dermatologist, proctologist, gynaecologist and psychiatrist.

Similar clinical situations are known as neurotic excoriations and prurigo. In these disorders, persistent generalized itch is the bitter complaint but all that one can ever find in neurotic excoriations are scratched spots or simple scratch marks. In prurigo the scratched areas are more raised due to the accompanying inflammation. There is no simple answer to these problems, but their recognition is important as it saves further investigation of the patient and inappropriate treatment.

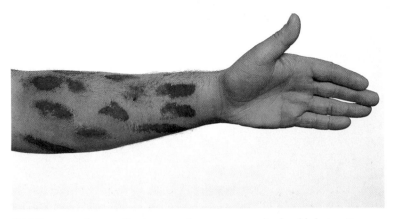

Odd linear erosions on the forearm of a young man. Such odd destructive lesions are likely to be self-induced.

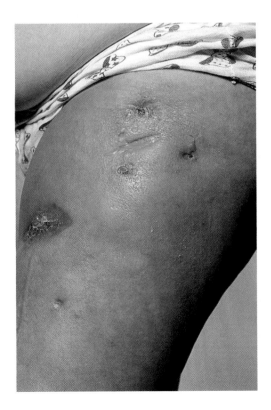

Artefactual lesions on the thigh of a young woman who suffered recurrent abscesses and sinuses. In this and other sites it was thought that she injected irritant material into her skin.

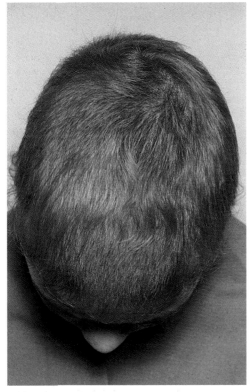

Trichotillomania. Many broken hairs are seen over this young woman's vertex. She later admitted to rubbing the area with her knuckles.

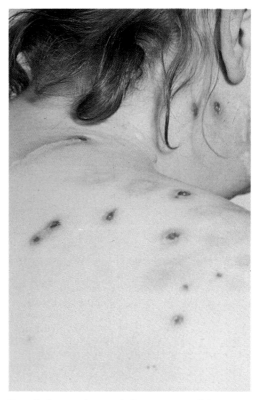

So-called neurotic excoriations occur mainly over the shoulders, face and arms, but may be seen elsewhere too.

PSYCHOSES AND THE SKIN

A further, more extreme link between skin and mind that needs discussion here is also uncommon but important to recognize. Schizophrenic patients and others with psychoses of various types may present with bizarre symptoms such as electric shocks all over the skin or of strange insects burrowing into it. I remember one dear old lady who visited my clinic on several occasions complaining of worms in her skin. She brought me an old-fashioned tin gramophone-needle box with rolled up bits of horn and scale in it which she had somehow dug out of her skin, believing them to be worms. Clearly, these individuals need urgent help from a department of psychiatry. Unfortunately these patients are difficult to help and psychiatrists are often unable to remove the delusional ideas.

DEPRESSION

A common and important relationship between the psyche and the skin is the very natural one of depression as a consequence of a persistently itchy and cosmetically disfiguring skin disease. We see each other via our skin. A healthy skin is intimately bound up with our own self-regard. When it is disfigured congenitally or deformed by disease we feel inferior – and this feeling is often magnified by the intuitive revulsion and unfeeling comments of many who come into social contact with sufferers from skin disease. This depression property of chronic skin disease should be recognized and handled with sympathy. If necessary, formal psychiatric consultation should be arranged.

MANAGEMENT

There is little that we can do to protect our patients from social, financial or emotional disasters. However, it is possible to reduce the consequences of these mishaps in the skin. Patient explanation of the relationship of the stress to the skin disorder is helpful and may be all that is required. On occasion it may be impossible for the patient to avoid an anticipated stress (exams or divorce, for example) and it may then be useful to prescribe some extra treatment to cope with the expected flare of the disorder. I have little faith in the remedial effects of the usually prescribed psychotropic drugs – such as valium – but am prepared to admit that some patients may be helped over a difficult period by their use.

When it is suspected that there is a serious psychiatric disorder underlying the skin problem, it is safer not to employ whatever amateur psychiatric skills you may possess, but to refer to a psychiatrist as soon as possible. I know of at least one patient who committed suicide after well-meaning but inefficient psychiatric management, when confronted with the accusation that she was causing the skin disease herself.

PRACTICAL POINTS

- No skin disease has been shown to be caused by stress, anxiety or depression, but several are often aggravated by them.
- Neurotic reactions can magnify dermatological symptoms and greatly extend their duration.
- Depression is often caused by disfiguring skin disease. These patients require extremely sensitive and sympathetic handling, and many benefit from specialist psychiatric help.
- In rare cases, skin lesions – such as inflammatory rashes and ulcers – can be self-induced (*Dermatitis artefacta*).

9

Sex and the skin

THE PSYCHOLOGICAL EFFECTS ON SKIN DISEASE ON SEX

The skin is an important bearer of secondary sexual characteristics and also serves as an organ of communication. When it is diseased, primitive fear and revulsion are experienced both by the sufferer and the unaffected observer. Although patients rarely state it during a consultation (there are few patients, or doctors, who feel uninhibited when discussing sexual problems, even in these comparatively enlightened times) one of their major concerns is the effect that their skin disorder will have on their sexual relationships. When the skin disease is persistent or recurrent – particularly with psoriasis, dermatitis and acne – this fear of loss of allure seems to cause much anxiety and depression.

This type of problem should be anticipated by the practitioner and gentle, tactful enquiry made about how the rash is affecting their sex lives. Sometimes it is useful to interview the partner as well as the patients, although whether they attend separately or together must depend on the particular circumstances of each case. Often all that is required is firm reassurance to the effect that the rash is not catching and need not affect their sexual activities in any way. If simple interview, discussion and explanation do not seem to provide the help necessary then assistance should be obtained from a dermatologist or psychiatrist, or both.

SEXUALLY TRANSMITTED DISEASES

The other aspect of the relationship between sexual activity and the skin concerns the broader present-day concept of sexually transmitted diseases.

Genital herpes

At present there is a pandemic of genital herpes. This disorder is very similar to ordinary herpes simplex occurring around the nose and mouth (cold sores), but the virus is slightly different antigenically. Herpes around the mouth (herpes virus type I) can also infect the genital region, but genital herpes (herpes virus type II) usually does not cause lesions elsewhere. Genital herpes not only affects the shaft of the penis or the vulva but can also produce lesions on the buttocks and thighs. The disorder is episodic as is facial herpes simplex, and when present can be very painful.

At the time of writing there is no way of preventing further attacks, although there are drugs – acyclovir (Zovirax) and famicyclovir (Famvir), available as an oral, topical or parenteral preparations – which do not 'cure' herpes but do seem to shorten the disease by 2–3 days and may decrease its severity. They do not decrease the chance of recurrence or increase the interval between episodes. For most patients with simple uncomplicated herpes simplex a topical preparation is all that is required. If the attack is particularly severe, acyclovir tablets 400 mg five times daily may also be given. Famicyclovir has recently been licensed but this drug does not appear to have any particular advantage over acyclovir. There is also an antiviral compound available – idoxuridine (Herpid) – which gives assistance to some patients if it is applied when there are premonitory symptoms and used 4-hourly during the day. The only other treatment available is to keep the affected area clean, dry and at rest during the attack. Although the disease may recur over a long period of time, it does not seem to persist for ever, and this fact may provide some reassurance for those affected.

Genital warts

Genital warts (see also pages 134 and 223) are also venereally transmitted. As with herpes infection, they are antigenically different from the virus that causes lesions elsewhere. When there are warts around the anal margin, homosexual contact is the likely cause.

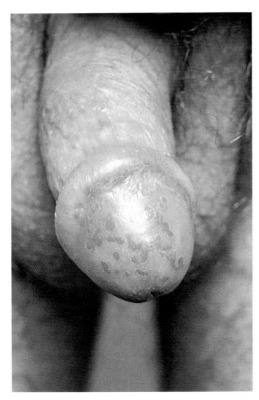

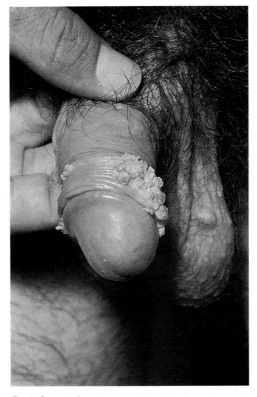

Herpes simplex affecting the glans penis in a young man. Eroded vesicles and other eroded areas can be seen.

Genital warts in a young man.

Podophyllin paints (tincture or collodion flex preparations), in concentrations ranging from 5 per cent to 20 per cent, cope with the majority of these lesions. The weaker concentrations are used at first and are painted accurately on the warts and allowed to remain there for some four to six hours. The genitalia are then bathed to get rid of the remaining podophyllin. This treatment is repeated weekly with increasing concentrations till the warts disappear. There is in addition a preparation (condyline) containing the active component of the podophyllin extract, the alkaloid podophyllotoxin. There is no special advantage in using this preparation. Podophyllin treatment can make the area very sore and the patient should be warned about this. It should be avoided in pregnancy because of potential teratogenicity. If podophyllin treatment is not successful then the warts may have to be removed by cautery and curettage, or cryotherapy.

Molluscum contagiosum

There is another viral disorder that can be transmitted by sexual contact. It is my impression that these virally induced lesions are more common now than they once were. They are easily recognized by their domed shape and central whitish plug which pops out if the lesion if squeezed. This procedure cures the lesion. The only other way of treating the disorder is with the various destructive techniques used for warts (see Chapter 22).

Vaginal candidiasis

This has become a common disorder presumably because of the widespread use of broad-spectrum antibiotics and the contraceptive pill. The infection can be passed to men, who then develop inflamed patches with pustules on the glans and the shaft of the

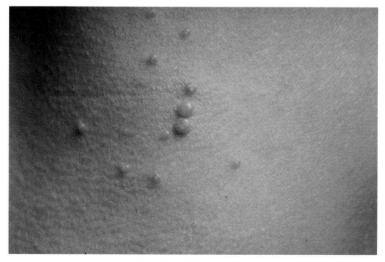

Molluscum contagiosum of the skin of the trunk in a young woman. Her boyfriend had similar lesions. The small pearly papules with a central depression are typical.

penis. The disease is easily treated in men with one of the imidazole group of drugs – eg, miconazole (Daktarin, Monistat) – but may be much more difficult to eliminate in women. Referral to a gynaecologist at an early stage is probably the best plan.

Scabies and pubic lice

The venereal nature of scabies and pubic lice is now well established. When treatment of these disorders is planned it is vital to include the sexual partners so that the disease is not passed back and forth, and further transmission to others is prevented.

PRACTICAL POINTS

● Sympathetic reassurance and explanation about the effects of nonvenereal disease on a patient's sex life may help to alleviate strong but often unexpressed anxieties.
● **Genital herpes**
There is no cure, but acyclovir (Zovirax) or famicyclovir (Famvir) may assist.
● **Genital warts**
Podophyllin paints should be the first-line treatment.
● **Candidiasis**
This is often cleared up using a pessary of one of the imidazole group of drugs or rhystatin.
● **Scabies and pubic lice**
Ensure both partners are treated concurrently.

10

Advice on cosmetics

BACKGROUND

Dermatologists are increasingly recognizing the importance of being able to provide adequate advice on the use of cosmetics. Questions concerning cosmetics frequently crop up in the practitioner's consulting room too.

It is not helpful to adopt a disapproving attitude to cosmetics. Regardless of your personal views they will continue to be used by a large proportion of the population. It should be remembered that the aims of dermatological treatments and cosmetics are similar in some respects – they both attempt to improve the appearance of the skin.

RASHES CAUSED BY COSMETICS

Most modern cosmetics are completely innocuous in that they rarely cause harm to the skin. They are far more often blamed than blameworthy. It is fairly common for a particular cosmetic to be held responsible for a rash which would in fact have appeared spontaneously, had the cosmetic not been used.

How to test

Occasionally one or other of the constituents of a particular cosmetic (lanolin, for example) will cause an allergic contact dermatitis in a patient, but this is surprisingly uncommon (see Chapter 34). A good plan when confronted with this sort of problem is to test the cosmetic in question by placing it on the uninvolved skin of the forearm or back for two days under an occlusive dressing. If no rash develops under the dressing then it is unlikely that the particular cosmetic is to blame. If you do this, remember to warn the patient about the possibility of a rash developing. Unfortunately this system is not totally foolproof and it is possible to obtain both false positive and false negative reactions. When there is any doubt or when any litigation is in question, or when it appears that a constituent of several cosmetics is causing a reaction, then it is as well to refer the patient to the dermatology clinic for full formal patch testing (see Chapter 38). In the majority of patients no reaction is produced at the site of application.

In some individuals close questioning will reveal that the problem experienced is entirely subjective; in other words the cosmetic causes stinging or some other type of discomfort, rather than a visible rash. This problem has never been adequately resolved

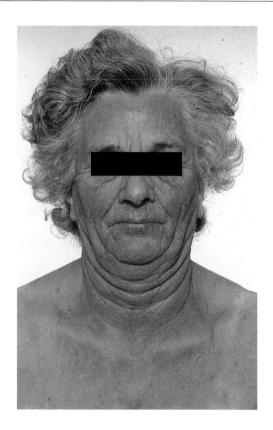

This woman suffered an allergic contact dermatitis to an emollient agent containing lanolin. It was also on her hands and forearm. Patch tests to lanolin were positive.

– undoubtedly some materials do cause this type of sensation quite consistently although we have no idea why. The only plan then is to use another cosmetic which by trial has been found to be more comfortable when applied.

'HYPOALLERGENIC' COSMETICS

Several companies market what are known (somewhat piously) as hypoallergenic cosmetics. These are supposed to contain only very 'safe' materials that do not cause skin problems. Opinions differ as to their usefulness. In general it appears that they are an unnecessary refinement for, as mentioned previously, nowadays most cosmetics contain only innocuous ingredients.

COSMETICS AND ACNE

Some of the thicker and oilier cosmetics seem to cause or precipitate acne lesions. If hair oils or greases are used and a fringe is allowed to dangle over the forehead, acne spots may occur on the forehead under the hair fringe. This has also been described with sun oils, with spots occurring on the chest and shoulders. When a youngster already has acne and asks what he or she should do about cosmetics, the reply should be sympathetic and could include the suggestion that lighter preparations are used and that heavier foundations are avoided.

There are some creams and lotions that are advertised for the treatment of acne spots and pimples which are also formulated to disguise the affected area. There is no particular harm in these and they may help some patients.

DEODORANTS AND ANTIPERSPIRANTS

Our obsession with hiding our natural body odours seems to be here to stay. Sticks, sprays and roll-on deodorants mostly contain aluminium and zirconium hexachlorhydrate, which stop the sweat glands functioning for some hours. Some also contain an antimicrobial such as hexachlorophane to reduce the bacterial flora and prevent odours from microbial degradation of sweat. These preparations rarely cause rashes. At one time there were antiperspirants that only contained zirconium which did cause an unpleasant form of inflammation, but these have been withdrawn.

Rarely, a fragrance or antimicrobial or some other component of the antiperspirant/deodorant will cause allergic contact dermatitis. If this appears to be the case, care should be taken that the patient does have a true allergic contact dermatitis and not some type of transient idiosyncratic intolerance. If the spray is applied to the arm or back of the area occluded with an adhesive plaster, the development of a patch of dermatitis at the site of application will make the diagnosis of allergic contact dermatitis much more likely.

Hyperhidrosis

Some unlucky individuals – particularly teenagers – sweat profusely from their axillae, feet, palms and face (hyperhidrosis) and find this a great nuisance and embarrassment. It can ruin footwear, blouses and shirts, and cause unpleasant smells and appearance. These body sites are most frequently affected, but other areas can be involved and it is quite common for only one or two sites to be affected. By the time sufferers consult a physician about their problem they have usually tried all the proprietary antiperspirants without success and are depressed about their problems.

There are stronger preparations available made especially for this disorder and one of these should be tried – aluminium chloride hexahydrate (Driclor), for example. If these do not work, systemic anticholinergic drugs such as propantheline bromide (ProBanthine) or poldine methylsulphate (Nacton) may sometimes help. Unfortunately the side-effects of a dry mouth and difficulties with accommodation are usually experienced before relief from the sweatiness is obtained.

It is probably wise to seek specialist advice sooner rather than later as there are a number of other approaches to treatment (including surgical, such as sympathectomy) which require considerable experience and are beyond the scope of this book.

COSMETIC CAMOUFLAGE

Large, deforming port-wine stains and ugly scars can be disguised by skilful use of special cosmetics formulated for the purpose. It is important that patients with these and

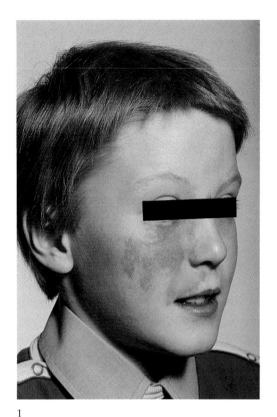
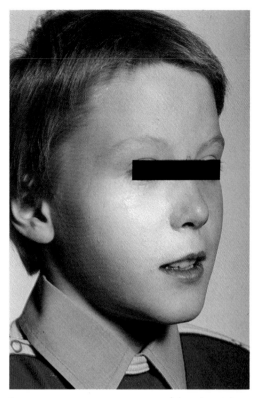

1

2

This sequence (1–4) shows the various stages of applications of a camouflage cream on a young man with a congenital port-wine stain on his cheek. With the help of a skilled cosmetician he has learnt how to disguise the condition very effectively.

similar problems are made aware of the possibility of this sort of help. Most large dermatology departments are fortunate to have the services of an expert in cosmetic camouflage and although there may be a waiting list it is probably wise to refer all individuals with deforming birthmarks and scars. It is now possible to remove or at least considerably improve vascular birthmarks – particularly port-wine stains – with the use of a laser. There are now many dermatology departments that have such equipment and skilled operators to use them. There are in addition many private clinics that offer a similar service. Laser treatment may also be helpful for patients with large melanocytic naevi and for tattoos but specialist advice should be obtained for these patients.

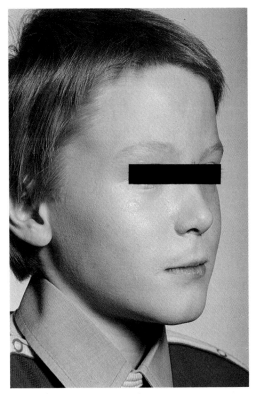

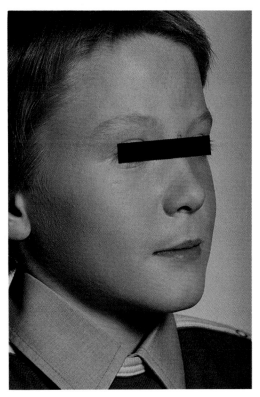

3   4

PRACTICAL POINTS

- Allergic contact dermatitis due to cosmetics is surprisingly rare.
- In straightforward cases, hypersensitivity to a particular cosmetic should be tested by placing it on uninvolved skin for two days under an occlusive dressing.
- Greasy cosmetics and sun oils can precipitate acne.
- Patients with deforming birthmarks and scars usually should be referred to a specialist cosmetician.
- Proprietary therapeutic/camouflage preparations may benefit some acne patients.
- If simple measures to control hyperhidrosis with antiperspirants are unsuccessful, specialist help is required.
- Laser treatment by experts may help patients with vascular birthmarks as well as those with tattoos and large melanocytic naevi.

11

Advice on sun and sun-lamps

THE ILL EFFECTS OF SUN EXPOSURE

Although most of us enjoy spending time in the sun, the sun's rays have damaging effects as well (see also pages 52–7). Unfortunately this is not yet sufficiently appreciated in the United Kingdom, although it is well understood in Australia, South Africa and the southern United States.

Sunburn

We all know about sunburn, or at least we think we do. It appears to be conventional wisdom that the fairer you are, the more easily you become sore in the sun, and that if you use suncream you prevent the burning effects of the sun. Unfortunately it is more complex than that! People of Celtic descent (including the darker ones), such as those who hail from Scotland, Ireland or Wales, seem to have a special predisposition to sun damage of all kinds.

People are particularly liable to sunburn between 11 am and 3 pm, and especially likely to suffer on high ground where there is little shade – on hills or while mountain climbing or skiing, for example – or on the beach or at sea. The sea, sand and snow are all good reflectors of the sun's energy, and where they are, there is usually little natural shade. It is also not often appreciated that it is easy to get sunburnt though thin clothing, and I have seen severe sunburn on areas protected by thin blouses and shirts.

Other skin disorders

Sunburn is not the only form of acute reaction caused by solar irradiation. Although some psoriasis sufferers may benefit from sun exposure, there are many skin disorders that are actually made worse by the sun – including lupus erythematosus and some types of dermatitis – and some skin disorders that are entirely dependent on exposure to the sun for their appearance – drug photosensitivities (see Chapter 13) and porphyria cutanea tarda, for instance. Polymorphic light eruption is a quite common skin disorder caused by sun exposure. It is seen on sun-exposed areas mainly in young and middle-aged women. Eczematous patches and itchy nodules appear a few hours after sun exposure.

Apart from these short-term considerations, the sun causes irreparable harm to the skin when there is exposure over long periods of time. It is a matter of the total dose of solar energy received, not the dose rate, although that too may be important in some

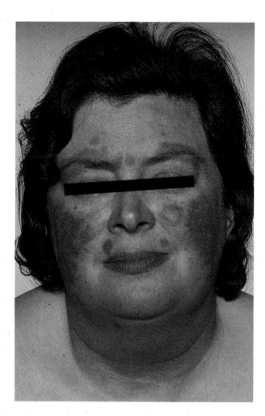

Lupus erythematosus aggravated by a period of sun exposure. This woman was aware that her condition was made worse by the sunlight but could not avoid exposure on this occasion.

Factors predisposing to solar injury

Constitutional
● 'Celtic-type' individuals. Fair-complexioned, blue-eyed people.
● Genetically determined solar sensitivity (eg, xeroderma pigmentosum).

Environmental
● Exposure to summer sun between 11 am and 3 pm.
● Exposure to highly reflective surroundings (eg, beach, snow, sea).
● Exposure to sun in equatorial and subequatorial zones.
● Exposure to sun at high altitude.

Failure of 'protection'
● Thin inadequate clothing.
● Inadequate sunscreen.
● Inadequate shade.

disorders. Wrinkling, the development of brown spots (senile lentigines), and a host of other skin changes are almost entirely due to long-term sun exposure. They are particularly obvious on the face, the neck, the backs of the hands and the forearms. Once again, fair-skinned individuals are particularly prone to these unpopular alterations to the skin

Some skin disorders caused by sun exposure

Short-term exposure
- Sunburn
- Drug-induced photosensitivities
- Polymorphic light eruptions
- Lupus erythematosus
- Porphyria cutanea tarda

Long-term exposure
- Wrinkling
- Senile lentigines
- Solar keratoses
- Basal cell carcinoma
- Squamous cell cancer
- Malignant melanoma

but they are also seen in darker-skinned people whom you might think should be better protected by their pigment.

Unfortunately these changes are not the only ones. Solar irradiation also causes cancer of the skin – squamous cell cancer and melanoma. Even in comparatively sunless Britain these disorders have become more prevalent since the advent of cheap holidays abroad; the average exposure to the sun of citizens in Britain is now approximately three times more than it was a decade ago. Apart from these frankly neoplastic lesions, numerous premalignant lesions appear in sun-damaged skin. These are known as solar keratoses and lentigines, and they are common in people who have spent long periods in hot sunny areas or have predominantly outdoor occupations.

PROTECTION FROM THE SUN

Sunscreens filter out the burning rays of the sun and are graded by what is known as a sun protection factor (SPF). This gives some indication of the increased period of time that can be spent in the sun without being burnt and refers to the individual's sun sensitivity. For example, if it takes two minutes for someone to turn red when unprotected, and he or she used a lotion with a SPF of 10, then theoretically he or she should be able to spend twenty minutes in the sun without looking like a lobster. Some individuals need preparations with a high SPF (15 or more); others need a less protective material. To all intents and purposes people with black or dark brown skin do not need as much protection from the sun, although even they can burn if they stay out for too long in intense sunshine. Fair-skinned blondes and redheads need maximal protection, as they are usually very sensitive.

Good sunscreens should protect against both the burning medium wave band ultra-violet radiation (UVR), known as UVB, and the long wave band UVR known as UVA. Although ordinary sunburn is not obvious after exposure to UVA, these rays can cause serious skin damage contributing to skin cancer formation as well as to wrinkling and senile lentigines. The stronger the sun's rays and the paler the skin of the individual the more protective the sunscreen should be.

As mentioned above, the SPF is a measure of the sunscreen's protection against burning UVB rays. It says nothing about its capacity to protect against UVA. A star rating system has been developed to describe the ratio of protection against UVB to that against UVA but is only used by some sunscreen manufacturers. The 'pack insert' should be read to learn about the protection offered by individual preparations.

The length of time for which sunscreens give protection depends on the way they cling to the skin surface. Swimming and abrasion from clothes and sand will take most of them off quite quickly, so that reapplication may be required. As to the choice of sunscreen, this must depend on its SPF and general cosmetic acceptability – a preparation that is not used because it is too greasy or smells bad is useless.

The best advice is moderation. There is nothing intrinsically beautiful about bronzed skin. It is worth relating that most cultures have prized a pale nonpigmented skin and regarded it as a sign of beauty in women. If people insist on exposing themselves to the hot sun, they should at least be advised to wear a broad-brimmed hat and to take the precaution of starting off slowly (a few minutes on the first day) and using an appropriate sunscreen.

SUN-LAMPS AND SUN BEDS

The above also applied to sun-lamps and sun beds. The more exposure obtained, the greater the damage. Even if one avoids being burned, there may be sufficient undetected injury to cause wrinkling or skin cancer to appear in later years.

In addition there are other potential hazards from sun-lamps when used in the home. I have seen several very unpleasant burns in patients who just did not appreciate how much irradiation they were receiving. There are also of course the ordinary electrical and mechanical hazards of such devices. I do not believe there is any place for sun-lamps in the home unless specifically recommended for the supervised treatment of particular skin diseases, such as psoriasis.

PRACTICAL POINTS

- It is the cumulative amount of sun exposure that causes long-lasting skin damage.
- The best advice to give on avoiding sunburn is:
  –Don't remain too long in the sun – stay out of the sun from 11 am to 3 pm.
  –Use a sunscreen with a high SPF and adequate protection against UVA.
  –Wear a broad-brimmed hat.
- Apart from sunburn and long term damage (including wrinkling and skin cancers) the sun causes a number of troublesome rashes e.g. polymorphic light eruption and drug photosensitivities.
- Sun-lamps and sun beds should not be recommended for home use, unless for supervised treatment of a specific skin disease.

12

Sport and the skin

BACKGROUND

Increasing time for leisure and sporting activities has produced a new set of problems for the skin. The practitioner is often asked to advise on how to protect the skin against sporting injury, and what kinds of sport should be avoided when suffering from a particular skin disorder. In addition, some kinds of rash are almost specific to some kinds of sport and these should be recognized and appropriately treated if required.

Protection against mechanical trauma is a prime function of the skin. Although only 0.012–0.02 mm thick, apart from the palms and soles, the stratum corneum is the first line of defence and protects efficiently against minor penetrating and abrasive injuries. Beneath the stratum corneum and epidermis is the dermal connective tissue which also has a very important protective function. It is both tough and elastic so that the skin is able to resist indentation and shearing forces. When these tissues are abnormal they are less able to resist injury.

PSORIASIS AND DERMATITIS

In both psoriasis and dermatitis the stratum corneum is brittle and crumbly, if present at all, so that the affected areas of skin are easily injured. This seems to be a problem mainly for youngsters with psoriasis, as the knees and elbows are often involved in this disease. The advice given must depend on the nature and extent of the rash and the stoicism and keenness of the individual concerned.

Patients with atopic dermatitis tend to develop infections of the skin and when this happens persistently after sporting injuries it may be as well to suggest that non-body-contact sports, such as tennis, may be preferable – at least until improvement occurs. When psoriasis or dermatitis affects the palms or soles extensively, vigorous activity of these parts (as in racquet sports) is to be avoided or else cracks may develop which delay resolution.

Problems due to corticosteroids

In patients with either dermatitis or psoriasis who have been using potent cortico-steroids, skin-thinning takes place. The blood vessels in the thinned skin are much more fragile than usual and bruises develop easily. Even worse, in extreme degrees of skin-thinning the skin may actually tear after relatively minor trauma. Such patients must be warned to avoid injury or else the most ghastly skin injuries can occur. Luckily, skin-thinning from corticosteroids is not usually a permanent problem; when use of the steroid cream is stopped, the thinning gradually rights itself, although it may take some months to do so.

DISORDERS OF CONNECTIVE TISSUE

There are some unusual congenital disorders of connective tissue in which broad and ugly scars form after injury – pseudoxanthoma elasticum, for example (see page 31). If patients with these disorders can be persuaded to restrict their sporting activities to noncontact sports, where they are unlikely to sustain significant injury to the skin, they will be grateful in the long term.

SKIN INFECTIONS

Another sporting health problem that frequently crops up concerns infections passed on as a result of shared changing facilities or skin-to-skin contact or just proximity to an affected individual. Sports such as wrestling, rugby, American football and swimming are particularly likely to serve as foci for skin infections of one sort and another.

Viral warts, ringworm infections and herpes simplex sores are notorious as sport-initiated infections. The close skin-to-skin contact of wrestlers occasionally results in what has come to be known as herpes gladiatorum! Less commonly impetigo and molluscum contagiosum are transmitted between competitors.

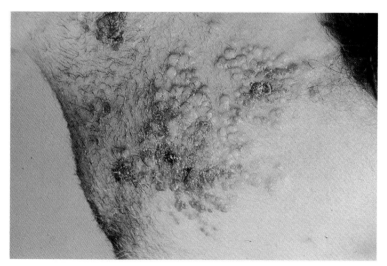

Quite severe herpes simplex of the neck in a rugby player, caught from skin contact with another player shedding the herpes virus.

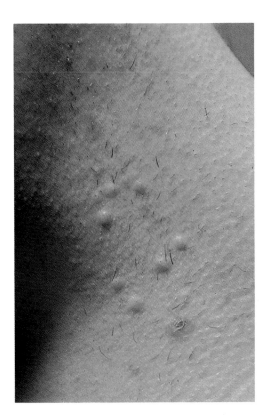

Molluscum contagiosum on a similar site and due to a similar cause as the picture on the previous page.

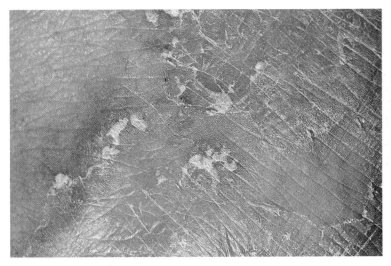

Ringworm of the sole of the foot. There was extensive scaling of both soles in this middle-aged man.

It is difficult to give the necessary stern and restrictive advice to patients that will prevent all these hazards. All these conditions are common, people often have them without even knowing (warts and ringworm infection, for example) and the effects of their transmission are usually trivial anyway. However, if the occasion arises those with active herpes simplex or impetigo lesions should be asked to desist from contact sports until their attack subsides. Similarly, if someone with active and scaling ringworm of the feet or body seeks advice they should be asked to avoid communal changing facilities and swimming until cured.

SWEAT RASHES

Miliaria

These skin lesions are caused by heavy sweating and sweat pore occlusion due to macerated soggy superficial skin. They occur particularly when it is hot and humid. The commonest form is the appropriately named miliaria crystallina in which tiny, thin-walled, shiny vesicles form. Deeper-set red itchy and/or painful papules (miliaria rubra) may also occur if the obstruction is deeper down in the sweat gland. They usually cause no symptoms and need no special treatment. Occasionally, deeper, more inflammatory

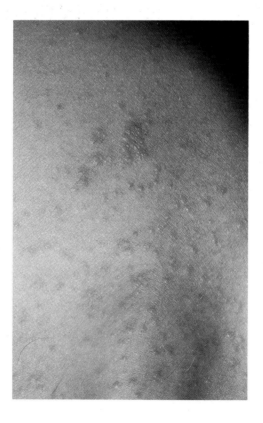

Miliaria. Numerous small white and pink-white papules appearing on the trunk of a young man in summertime.

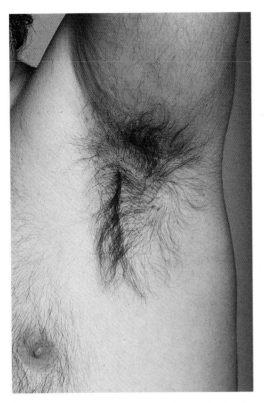 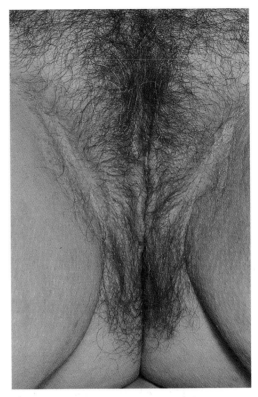

Intertrigo caused by vigorous sporting activities in a slightly overweight patient.

This young woman was somewhat overweight and developed her intertrigo while playing several matches in a tennis tournament.

Sport-related skin problems

- **Viral warts**
- **Ringworm** } Close-contact and 'communal-changing-room' sports
- **Herpes simplex**
- **Miliaria**
- **Intertrigo** } Vigorous sports in hot and humid conditions
- **Haematoma**　　　　Body-contact and racquet sports
- **Blisters, callosities**　Racquet sports, athletics, rowing, running team-games
- **Sunburn**　　　　　Winter sports, yachting, outdoor summer sports
- **Frostbite**　　　　Mountaineering
- **Chilblains**　　　　Sea swimming, yachting, horse-riding
- **Otitis externa**　　Swimming

lesions develop, and these are itchy and sore. Sufferers from these sweat rashes need to be kept cool and may also need local symptomatic treatment – cooling and astringent lotions such as witch hazel may be helpful.

Intertrigo

Sore red rashes may develop in the major flexures of heavily built sportsmen and -women when the weather is hot and damp. These patches are not due to ringworm although they arise at the same sites and are similar in appearance. Some call this condition 'sweat rash' or intertrigo, while others prefer 'seborrhoeic dermatitis'. It is probably due to a combination of mechanical injury from the rubbing of clothes on skin surfaces (the perpetually wet horny layer is weaker than normal) and mild infections (due to overgrowth of the normal skin bacteria). At times it may be very itchy because the inflamed skin develops an eczematous reaction. The clue to distinguishing it from ringworm is that this intertrigo-type rash is symmetrical and reaches up into the apices of the groin.

Stopping all vigorous exercise and staying cool usually clears it up in a day or two. Sometimes a weak, nonirritant antimicrobial cream – such as miconazole (Daktarin, Monistat) – may be required for the more severely affected (see Chapter 28). If there is eczema present as well, a combination of an antimicrobial with hydrocortisone – such as Daktacort – is helpful.

SPORT-INDUCED LESIONS

Some sports produce characteristic lesions on the skin and these need to be recognized as they are no longer uncommon and explanations and reassurance may be necessary.

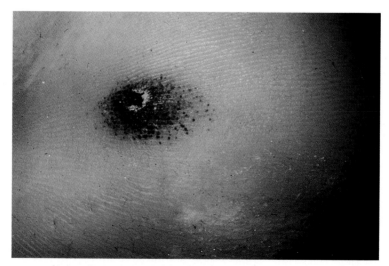

Black dots aggregated like this and appearing on the heels are the result of a shearing injury and are often found in squash players.

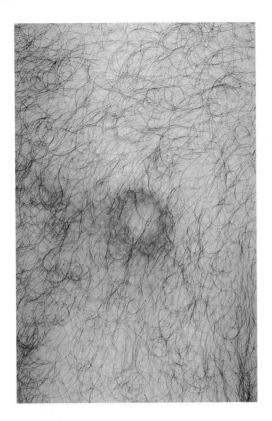

Injury from a squash ball produces a rather characteristic lesion, with a paler area at the centre and a ring of erythema.

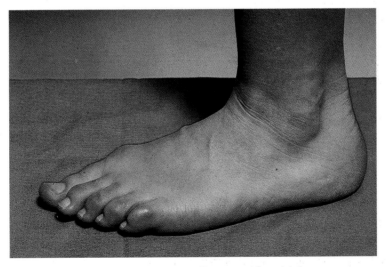

Chilblains. The area over the toes is swollen, mauvish and itchy.

The rise in the popularity of squash has resulted in a spate of consultations for odd areas of black-dot-type lesions on the heels. These are the result of the sharp turns required in this game which produce shearing stresses on the skin of the soles.

Being hit by a squash ball is momentarily painful but results in a characteristically colourful contusion that lasts several days. Curiously the centre of these is quite pallid while the periphery of the bruise is at first merely suffused; later it takes on the usual hues of a fading contusion. Apart from callosities on the hand holding the racket there are no other characteristic skin lesions of squash of which I am aware.

Blisters occur on the palms and soles when there is unaccustomed trauma. Usually they require no treatment other than being kept clean and covered. Callosities are seen in a variety of other anatomical sites in sportsmen dependent on what causes friction against what and for how long. They rarely cause symptoms save when the tissues beneath become inflamed for one reason or another. It is doubtful whether any application can actually harden the skin – despite the liberal use of surgical spirit in some sporting circles.

SUNBURN

One category of ills to which the sportsman is prone is due to solar exposure (this is described in more detail in Chapter 11). Winter sports are not exempt from the problems of overexposure to the sun, which are common due to the high altitude and the reflection of light from the snow, although for obvious reasons the site of solar injury is usually restricted to the face.

Yachting, surfing and beach games may lead to sunburn, as, of course, may any other summer outdoor activity. Golf seems to be a particular problem for some – particularly the bald fair-skinned individual. The game seems so addictive that advice about 'taking care' is rarely heeded. Those who burn easily and do not tan readily should be warned of the long-term dangers of repeated sun exposure and given advice on sunscreens and other types of protection. Mostly this applies to fair-haired, blue-eyed individuals, but darker types may also suffer sunburn.

THE COLD AND DAMP

The cold and damp can also cause skin disorders in sporting types. The extreme case is frostbite in mountaineers, but lesser degrees of cold injury are more likely to be seen by practitioners, especially in this era of keen joggers and marathon runners.

Chilblains are one common type of mild cold injury and may be seen in sea swimmers or yachtsmen. Sometimes they occur in unexpected areas of the skin, particularly in plump young women who ride horses. Mauve, swollen patches can appear over the thighs and buttocks in these youngsters.

Otitis externa

Swimmers sometimes develop sore, inflamed ear canals. This otitis externa can become persistent and very troublesome if swimming is continued during attacks. When it develops acutely swimming must stop and an antibiotic (penicillin, ampicillin or tetracycline)

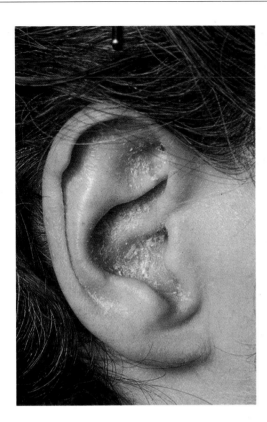

Otitis externa. This can be a real problem for keen swimmers.

should be given systemically. After the acute attack there should be a gap of several days before swimming is allowed. Again, the use of earplugs may be advisable. If the condition recurs on several occasions the patient should be referred to a specialist.

Jogger's nipple

No account of sporting injury to the skin would be complete without mention of this minor gem. It results from abrasion of the nipple against the vest, particularly if this is made of rough or fluffy material. Jogger's nipple is predominantly a problem of men, as women are protected by bras. The condition causes soreness and cracking – even bleeding. It can be minimized by the use of vaseline before running.

PRACTICAL POINTS

- In view of the ever-increasing number of participants in sport, practitioners would do well to familiarize themselves with the treatments for the wide range of sport-related skin conditions.
- Topical steroids cause skin-thinning when used for long periods and thus may cause problems in body-contact sports.
- Sport-playing patients with infected dermatitis or psoriasis, or active herpes simplex or impetigo lesions, should be advised not to participate in body-contact sports until the infection has cleared up.
- It may be necessary to prescribe a weak, nonirritant antimicrobial or antimicrobial/weak corticosteroid combination cream for severe cases of intertrigo.
- Acute otitis externa in swimmers should be treated with a systemic antibiotic and swimming should cease for a few days.

13

Drug-induced skin disease

BACKGROUND

The constant stream of new drugs and modifications of older ones dictates that we relearn clinical pharmacology every five years or so. It also ensures that the profile of drug-induced skin disease is constantly changing.

Penicillin-induced urticaria was more common when penicillin was one of the very few antibiotics available. Even the morbilliform eruption due to ampicillin is less common now than it was ten years ago. Fixed drug eruptions were more often seen when phenolphthalein was a commonly used laxative.

Because of these shifting clinical sands the only way to avoid being caught with one's diagnostic pants down is to maintain a high level of suspicion. Always ask patients with odd rashes 'What pills, medicines or injections are you taking?' Sometimes it will be necessary to badger patients a little on this point, as they often don't think of their aspirins, laxatives or vitamin pills as drugs.

Tests

Unfortunately there are no reliable ways of proving by a laboratory test that a particular drug caused a particular rash. The best way is still to 'challenge' the patient by readministering the drug, but it may not always be possible to do this – especially outside hospital. If there has been a life-threatening or very severe reaction (or suspected reaction) then clearly it would be quite improper to readminister the drug. The decision can be difficult, and specialist advice will probably be required.

Mimics

A very large number of drugs can cause some type of skin disorder. Drugs can cause nail, hair and pigmentation problems as well as rashes. It used to be said that syphilis was the great mimic, but this attribution now more correctly belongs to drug-induced skin disease. Although there are often physical features that will bring to mind the likelihood of a drug rash, it is quite common to see a drug-induced eruption similar in appearance to that of a spontaneously occurring skin disease such as lichen planus or lupus erythematosus.

It is not possible in a book of this type to catalogue all drug reactions, or to describe individual ones in any great detail. The aims of this chapter are to alert the practitioner to the frequent occurrences of this kind of skin disorder, to indicate the ranges of reactions possible and to advise on the best action to take if a drug rash occurs.

EXANTHEMATIC RASHES

Drug-induced rashes tend to be generalized but need not necessarily be so. Probably the commonest type of eruption is the exanthematic type. This breaks out suddenly and can look like measles or rubella. It is often quite itchy and there may be some generalized unwellness with its appearance.

Many kinds of drug can produce this sort of rash, including diuretics, nonsteroidal anti-inflammatory drugs (NSAIDs), psychotropics and antibiotics. If the offending drug is stopped the rash goes away in a few days. There seems little point in giving antihistamines to these patients – all these drugs will do in these circumstances is cause some drowsiness. To relieve the itch, mentholated oily calamine lotion is as good as anything I know.

URTICARIAL RASHES

Urticarial rashes are also common (see Chapter 34). These are also generalized but the individual lesions come and go at different sites, lasting a few hours only at any one site. Rarely this can be very severe with deep swellings of the affected areas. The life-threatening syndrome of oedema of the tongue and throat with generalized collapse is luckily very unusual now, but still can occur after injections of penicillin. Urticarial rashes may not stop immediately after the drug responsible is withdrawn.

The commonest offender is in fact penicillin but many other drugs, including morphine alkaloids, can cause urticaria. Aspirin, and all those analgesic preparations that contain it, can also cause urticarial rashes – probably through a nonallergic mechanism.

Giving antihistamines by mouth is of use for this condition and may give considerable relief. If the administration of antihistamines and the stopping of all other drugs do not control the appearance of the lesions and these continue in large numbers the opinion of an expert should be sought.

ULTRAVIOLET SENSITIVITY

Some drugs can sensitize the skin so that it reacts abnormally to the sun's ultraviolet light. The sulphonamides, the phenothiazines and the tetracyclines are long-established culprits as far as these photosensitivity reactions are concerned. Demeclocycline (Deteclo, Ledermycin) sometimes has the curious effect of sensitizing the nail tissues so that light exposure causes separation of the nail plate from the nail bed (photo-onycholysis). Chlorpromazine (Largactil) can cause a strange purple discolouration of the exposed skin in subjects given the drug over a long period. The drug given for cardiac arrhythmias – amiodarone – not uncommonly causes a type of photosensitivity in which exposed skin develops an odd slate-grey pigmentation. Generally, light-induced rashes are not difficult to detect as the eruption is, for the most part, confined to the directly light-exposed area.

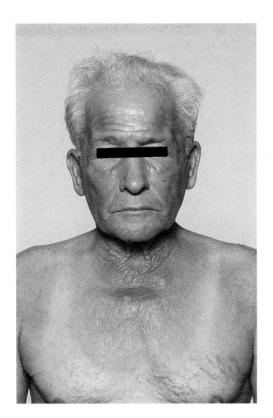

A photosensitivity reaction. This man was given tetracycline for his chronic bronchitis and developed a rash in the light-exposed areas. Notice how the redness is confined to the areas not covered by his vest – he was a keen gardener.

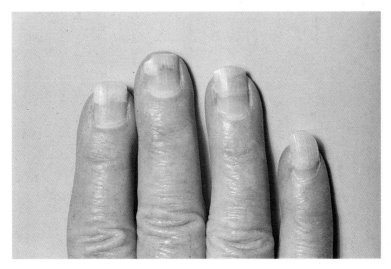

This man also had a phototoxic effect from taking demethylchlortetracycline. The separation of the nail from the nail-plate is known as photo-onycholysis and may be seen in other drug-induced photosensitivities.

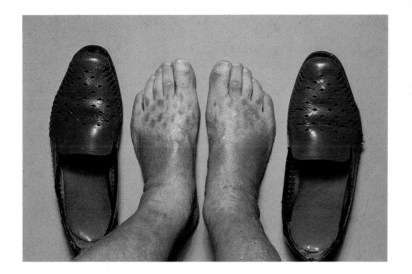

This man was easily persuaded that his rash was due to light exposure, once the relationship between the spots on his feet and the holes in his shoes was pointed out! His sensitivity to light might have been caused by one of the sulphonamides.

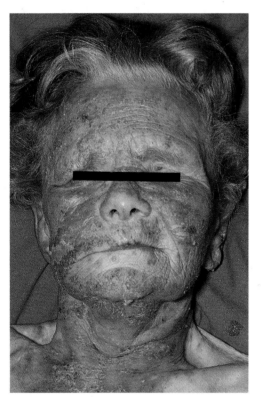

Toxic epidermal necrolysis can be an extremely severe disease and has a high mortality. This woman died despite nursing in an intensive care unit for ten days. Her skin and mucosae were extremely inflamed. The drug responsible was thought to be one of the nonsteroidal anti-inflammatory agents (NSAIDs) given for her arthritis.

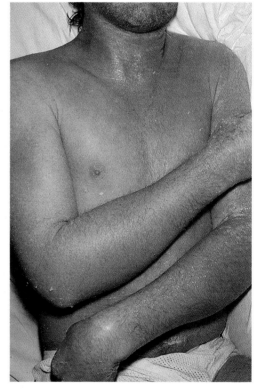

Exfoliative dermatitis in a young man given carbamazepine (Tegretol). When the drug was stopped his eruption gradually improved.

Most patients with drug-induced light sensitivities improve rapidly after stopping the drug responsible. They will also improve – though less quickly – if further light exposure is prevented or at least considerably reduced. As confirmation of the diagnosis is important and may need complex tests, including light tests, it is probably best to refer patients with this type of reaction for specialist opinion. Unfortunately there are a small group of patients whose light sensitivity does not rapidly remit after the drug responsible is stopped. These patients are said to suffer from the 'persistent light reaction' and because of their intolerance of even minimal amounts of light exposure, they constitute a very serious problem of management.

SEVERE REACTIONS

The severest types of drug reaction do not spontaneously improve soon after stopping the drug responsible and almost all patients will require admission to hospital. The reactions include erythema multiforme, toxic epidermal necrolysis and exfoliative dermatitis. The first two are blistering or erosive-type skin disorders and have an appreciable mortality; the affected patient is often extremely sick and requires urgent and expert attention. Anti-inflammatory drugs, antithyroid drugs, oral hypoglycaemic agents, gold injections and diuretics are among those agents that can cause these severe reactions.

PRACTICAL POINTS

Skin reaction	Main drug types responsible
● Exanthemic rash	Antibiotics, antirheumatics, diuretics, psychotropics
● Urticarial rash	Aspirin-containing analgesics, penicillin, morphine alkaloids
● Ultraviolet sensitivity	Phenothiazines, sulphonamides and tetracyclines
● Erythema multiforme Toxic necrolysis Exfoliative dermatitis	Antirheumatics, antithyroids, diuretics, gold injections, oral hypoglycaemics
● Blistering disorders	Penicillamine, captopril, frusemide, nalidixic acid.

14

Bites and stings

BACKGROUND

We share the world with a host of hungry and/or angry creatures both large and small. They nip, bite, scratch and sting either in defence or to obtain nourishment when they encounter human skin. In many instances attack only occurs when the creature is disturbed, presumably as a pre-emptive defence mechanism.

Potential aggressors range from tigers to ticks and to cover the entire subject here would be impossible. Some aspects are covered elsewhere (see page 49 and Chapter 25); here, my main aims are to describe the more common varieties of bites and stings encountered in Europe and to discuss their management. I will not discuss dog or snake bites as neither are really dermatological problems although skin infection, swelling and inflammation and ischaemic necrosis of the skin may result from these.

COMMON SORTS OF INSECT BITE

Bites from pet ectoparasites

Most of us have experienced flea bites and put up with them as an almost inevitable consequence of keeping furry cuddly pets. Virtually all flea bites are due to bites from cat and dog fleas and not due to the 'human' flea known as *Pulex irritans*. They are usually easily recognized as red spots 1–3 mm in diameter – often with central puncta at the apices of the papules. Flea bites tend to occur on the lower legs and to occur in crops. They are particularly frequent after occupation of property that once housed pets but stayed empty for a while. Human vibrations seem to activate the nymphs in flea eggs so that new inhabitants are attacked voraciously.

Flea bites seem to cause no major harm but are annoying and cause irritation. They may become infected when scratched. Treatment is directed to relieving the irritation and identifying the source. Spraying affected pets and carpets with anti-flea powders containing pyrethrum alkaloids is usually sufficient to remove the nuisance.

Dog scabies looks rather like human scabies (see page 153) but because the mite isn't adapted to man it only causes the rash where the retainer is in close contact with the patient. Another mite affecting dogs, known as *Chyletiela parasitovorax*, can also cause itchy rash in humans.

The actual bites themselves are itchy and these symptoms improve with 0.5 per cent menthol in oily calamine cream used when required. Antihistamine creams and weak corticosteroids may also give some relief.

Wasp and bee stings

The warmer summers of recent years in the UK have resulted in mini plagues of these creatures and an increase in the numbers of stings from them. They are always painful but not often dangerous. The only hazard is the development of immediate hypersensitivity and an anaphylactic reaction on being stung subsequently. Rarely, the resulting

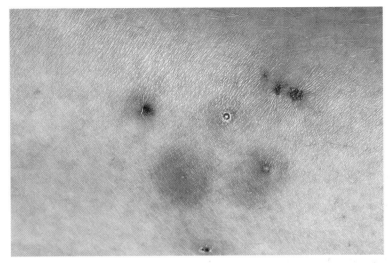

Flea bites on the leg.

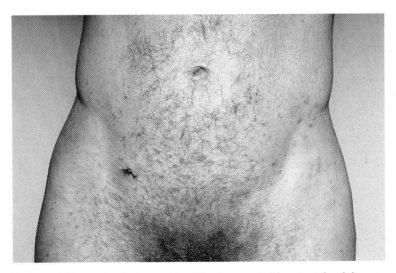

Rash on abdomen due to dog scabies. The dog was held against the abdomen during a 'petting session'.

shock, hypotension and bronchospasm causes death. Desensitization is certainly possible and should be recommended for sensitized individuals. Only those who are experienced in the technique of desensitization, know the dangers and take all precautions should undertake such prophylactic treatment. Antihistamines by mouth alone provide some relief and may also be used parenterally for patients with mild generalized reactions. For those with more severe reactions intramuscular promethazine (or other antihistamines) may be helpful. Severe respiratory symptoms and/or collapse require urgent treatment with subcutaneous adrenaline (1:1000), intravenous hydrocortisone and attention to the possible need for parental fluids and a tracheostomy. Self-injection kits containing adrenaline should be carried by those known to be hypersensitive to wasp or bee stings.

Mosquito bites

Mosquitoes are unpleasant little creatures that spread disease and cause annoyance and discomfort worldwide. Not all suck blood but many of those that do can spread such diseases as malaria, yellow fever and filariasis. Apart from the spread of disease the 'bites' they produce are usually intensely itchy and may be painful. Quite large areas of redness and swelling are by no means uncommon and in some cases large blisters develop. The acute symptoms last a few days and then gradually fade away. Scratching the lesions can result in skin infections including impetigo and ecthyma.

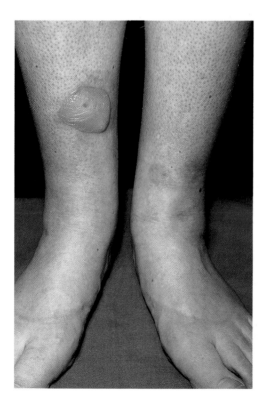

Large blister on lower legs due to mosquito bite.

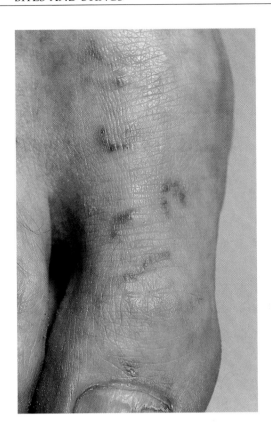

Larva migras on foot in individual returning from Kenya.

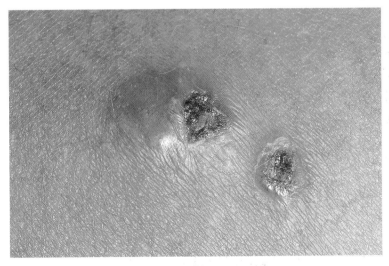

Human myiasis.

MISCELLANEOUS PROBLEMS

Gnats and ants can produce minor stings which itch and/or burn but these usually amount to no more than a minor annoyance and there is rarely much of a visible reaction to these insects. Ladybirds can also produce minor stings. Some hairy caterpillars can produce unpleasant inflammatory reactions just by brushing up against them.

Tick bites are uncommon but are distinguished by the creatures burrowing down into the skin, making them extremely difficult to remove. The 'deer tick' can spread Lyme disease by its bite. This can be treated either by mouth or topically with thiabendazole.

Bed bugs (*Limex lectularius*) should really be called 'old house' bugs because they live in the nooks and crannies of old buildings rather than beds. They usually crawl out of the woodwork at night and take a walk on whatever limb of whoever is available. This nocturnal strolling explains the series of bites occurring in a straight line. These can be quite large and unpleasantly inflamed.

Itchy rashes in a curious serpiginous pattern develop on the foot or buttocks in individuals returning from Africa and the Caribbean who have been in contact with wet sand or moist soil containing larval forms of dog hookworm. This can be treated either by mouth or topically with thiabendazole.

Some 'bot flies' lay eggs in human wounds and ulcers or, rarely, in intact skin. This unpleasant form of parasitism, known as myiasis, is mainly seen in sheep and cattle in the UK but can rarely occur in man as well.

Problems for bathers

Apart from the great white shark there are many biting and stinging creatures out in the sea. The most frequent problem is being stung by jellyfish tentacles. Other problems around the shores of north-west Europe include itchy rashes from algal blooms and skin infections from sea water, contaminated with bacteria. Rarely, stepping onto a sea urchin spine may cause inflammation in the foot and in warmer waters further south shocks from electric eels and serious stings from the spines of weaver fish are unusual hazards.

PRACTICAL POINTS

- Flea and mite bites are a common nuisance resulting from contact with animals infested with these ectoparasites.
- Mosquito bites can cause intense irritation and are sometimes infected by the scratching caused. They can spread serious diseases such as malaria and filariasis in tropical areas.
- Bee and wasp stings are painful but not generally dangerous unless the patient has become sensitive to the sting, in which case they can develop a severe anaphylactic reaction.

PART TWO: TREATMENT

15

Treatment of atopic dermatitis

Atopic dermatitis is one of the more intractable and distressing skin disorders and needs all the skill and patience that the practitioner (and dermatologist) can muster. The persistent itch, sleeplessness and anxiety that this causes require sympathy and understanding.

IDENTIFY THE AGGRAVATING FACTORS

The first thing to determine is whether there are any obvious aggravating factors that the patient encounters.

Diet

Do particular foodstuffs make the condition worse? The argument about cow's milk has not been settled as yet but if either patient or parent is convinced that milk makes the condition worse then a trial should be made of a milk-exclusion diet.

The same is true of any other foodstuff that is accused. Some find that eggs or fruit bring on attacks or aggravate the condition. If strict avoidance of the suspected allergen does little for the disease then there is not much point in persisting, but it is certainly worth making the attempt at exclusion from the diet. If dietetic treatments are contemplated it is important to 'build in' as much objectivity and absence of bias into a preliminary trial as possible. An unequivocal negative is just as important as a positive. When suspected foodstuffs are subjected to trials which are evaluated critically it is quite uncommon for the suspicion to be sustained.

Clothing

Woollen clothes are tolerated badly by many atopics and now that there are cheap smooth synthetic garments there seems little point in persisting with the older fluffier ones.

Stress and anxiety

Although stress or anxiety do not cause the disease they certainly seem capable of making it worse. The accounts of children's dermatitis getting worse before examinations at school are too frequently heard to be ignored.

However, although recognition of this sort of problem is important, it is much more difficult to know what to do about it. The worsening of the dermatitis before exams or some other stressful event should be anticipated and if possible guarded against. If the worsening that stress produces cannot be prevented, it is probably better to put up with it than avoid the stress. Avoidance of this type of stress inevitably generates other problems – and examinations are still important! (see also Chapter 8).

When children scratch their way through the night and cry with the discomfort it inevitably causes anxiety and guilt in the parents. Eventually this may lead to a very unpleasant atmosphere within the family where no-one sleeps and everyone is bad-tempered. In these circumstances a temporary separation of the affected child from the family may be the best answer. If necessary a few days of intensive treatment in hospital can be arranged.

TREATMENT

Emollients

Patients with atopic dermatitis have dry skin even when they don't have much obvious inflammation. The dry skin is itchy and uncomfortable and if left untreated predisposes to more dermatitis. It is important that patients are taught to keep their skins moist and supple. They should use some emollient preparation as often as this is necessary for their comfort (see also Chapter 17). The particular emollient chosen should be the one that they find most helpful and least unpleasant to use. The most efficient emollients contain more white soft paraffin but these tend to be the most greasy. Apart from emollient applications they should use a soap substitute with an emollient effect. Bath oils are also helpful in many patients (eg, Oilatum bath emollient or Balneum).

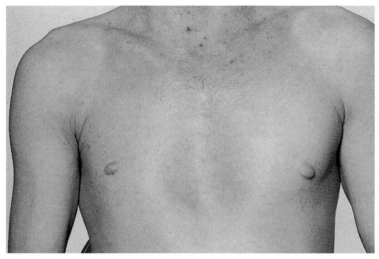

Typical atopic dermatitis is frequently accompanied by dry scaling skin (xeroderma). This causes considerable discomfort in some patients.

Topical corticosteroids

For the dermatitic patches themselves the mainstays of treatment are the topical corticosteroids (see also Chapter 27). The least potent preparations that produce improvement should be chosen. Atopic dermatitis tends to last for some years and there are serious dangers from the absorption of the corticosteroid if its application is continued. For this reason corticosteroids should only be used when the dermatitis is active.

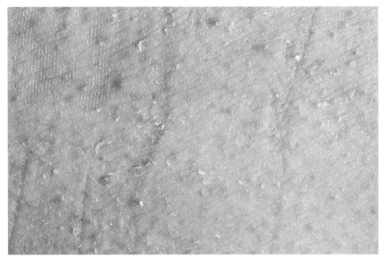

Dry skin in atopic dermatitis.

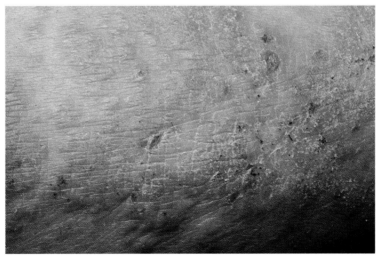

Chronic persistent lichenified dermatitis. This type of dermatitic rash frequently benefits from applications containing tar.

Hydrocortisone preparations are the most suitable but other weak corticosteroids, such as clobetasone butyrate (Eumovate) or 1 per cent hydrocortisone and 10 per cent urea (Alphaderm), may also be used. More potent corticosteroids should only be used for stubborn areas if needed, and then only for short periods.

Traditional treatments

Some of the older remedies should be given a chance. Weak tar preparations quite often exert a beneficial effect, especially on the more persistent thickened patches. Even zinc cream and oily calamine lotion can help some patients.

Bandaging may be helpful if it's a matter of preventing the creams or ointments from soiling the clothes or bed linen. They should not be used to restrain a child – the frustration of not being able to scratch an itch is worse than the damage to the skin caused by scratching.

Antihistamines

There is no place for topical antihistamines in the treatment of atopic dermatitis. They are not antipruritic in eczema and may irritate or even cause sensitization reactions. Systemic antihistamines of the older type are often prescribed to allay the itching. In fact the antihistamines seem to have very little effect on itching when pharmacological tests are made but agents such as dipthenhydramine, trimeprazine and chlorpheniramine cause drowsiness and relieve symptoms in this way. Newer non-sedating antihistamines such as terfenadine are not of much help to patients with atopic dermatitis.

PATIENTS' ORGANIZATIONS

Finally, a word about the National Eczema Society of Great Britain. This organization is to be strongly recommended for chronic dermatitis sufferers and their families. It provides practical support and brings home to the patient that many others are similarly affected – which seems to help.

Most large urban areas of Britain have a branch. Branch locations can usually be obtained from the local department of dermatology, but if difficulty is experienced the head office should be contacted (see Useful Addresses, page 241).

PRACTICAL POINTS

● Aggravating factors should be identified and, where possible, avoided. These include:
  –Stress and anxiety
  –Household items (dust, pets, etc)
  –Clothing (woollens)
  –Diet (cow's milk, eggs, fish, fruit, etc).
● If the family situation is extremely tense a spell as a hospital in-patient may be helpful.
● Treatments include:
  –Emollients
  –Topical corticosteroids (weakest possible)
  –Weak tars
  –Zinc cream
  –Oily calamine lotion
  –Systemic antibiotics
  –Systemic antihistamines.

16

Treatment of hand dermatitis

BACKGROUND

Hand dermatitis is one of the commonest causes of disability. When the palms and fingers are affected by dermatitis the skin is sore and may be cracked, preventing proper hand movements. In addition the scaling and oozing from vesicles make it difficult to perform 'clean' tasks.

DIAGNOSIS

The first step in management is to make a definitive diagnosis. Referral to a department where the appropriate tests can be carried out is probably wise for those patients in whom it is clear that the disorder is going to persist for some time.

With hand dermatitis, as with so many categories of skin disease, it is important to rule out such potentially curable disorders as ringworm and allergic contact dermatitis, after which the somewhat intellectually unsatisfying but pragmatic diagnosis of constitutional hand dermatitis may be made. Many patients with this problem are now thought to be suffering from a type of atopic dermatitis. Let us assume this point has been reached.

MANAGEMENT

Protecting the hands

To prevent further damage to the skin and to permit both rest and the application of treatments it may be best to recommend a period off work early on in the disorder (see Chapter 5). Certainly, manual work with abrasive or chemically irritant materials should be discouraged until the condition has completely resolved. This applies to housework too, although it is less easy to comply with this instruction. A compromise may have to be reached in which clean dry work is done only and gloves are worn when there is any type of potentially injurious activity planned. The work gloves I recommend are made of PVC and are cotton lined. Most patients find them quite satisfactory for work and better than rubber gloves. If these are not easily available, ordinary rubber gloves worn with cotton inner gloves will suffice.

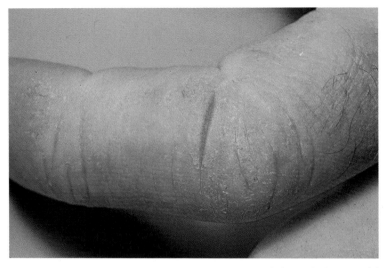

Chronic dermatitis of the hands often produces fissured skin, which is painful and disabling.

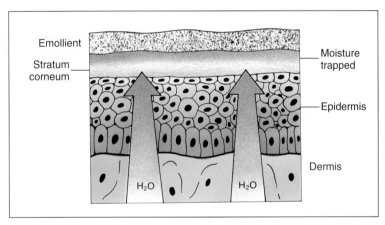

This diagram illustrates the action of emollients on the skin.

When the dermatitis begins to improve with treatment, the skin will still require some time before full recovery occurs, so care should continue to be taken to avoid further damage to the skin.

Emollients

Some toilet soaps are mildly irritating and so it has become usual practice to recommend some type of soap substitute or emollient cleansing agent (such as emulsifying ointment

BP, E45 wash cream, Neutrogena or Oilatum soap). They tend to prevent the drying out effect that some soaps have and, by helping hydration of the stratum corneum, may help maintain the horny layer in a flexible state.

Application of emollients plays an important role in the treatment plan. Emollients not only smooth the skin, make the horny layer more pliable and temporarily relieve irritation and discomfort, but they also have a small but definite intrinsic anti-inflammatory effect.

The best emollient is the one that the patient will actually use because he or she finds that it makes the condition more comfortable and does not offend any of the senses. White soft paraffin (Vaseline) is quite effective but because it is greasy is not tolerated by many. When there are fissured areas, 2 per cent salicylic acid in white soft paraffin applied at night is quite effective in promoting healing.

Topical corticosteroids

The above may be all that is required for some patients, although the majority will need an anti-inflammatory corticosteroid application as well. The most appropriate topical corticosteroid is the least potent one that has an adequate therapeutic effect (see Chapter 27). Generally, either a preparation containing hydrocortisone, clobetasone butyrate (Eumovate), or hydrocortisone with urea (eg, Alphaderm) is adequate. Diluted potent topical corticosteroids such as quarter strength Betnovate (Betnovate RD) may be suitable but the factor of dilution may be much greater than the effective reduction in potency.

Tar

When the dermatitic process is persistent and there is considerable skin thickening and scaling one of the tar-containing preparations may be helpful – though it is difficult to

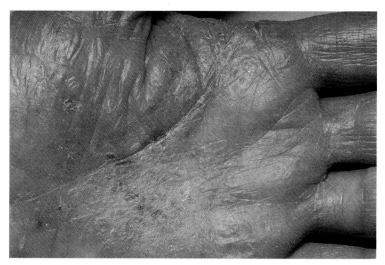

Chronic dermatitis of the hands. Such patients often benefit from the use of preparations containing tar.

persuade patients to use these on their hands. Cotton gloves worn at night over the tar preparation are generally acceptable. Some newer proprietary tars (eg, Clinitar cream and Alphosyl cream) are not quite so unpleasant to use and stain, sting and smell less than the traditional agents.

Astringent/antiseptic solutions

If there are oozing and vesicular patches then some benefit can be obtained by bathing the hands three or four times per day in one of the mild astringent and/or antiseptic solutions. I often employ very diluted potassium permanganate (1:8000 concentration) for this purpose.

PRACTICAL POINTS

● The patient should be advised to refrain from domestic and professional activities that involve contact with abrasive or chemically irritant materials or detergents.
● If this is impractical, cotton-lined protective gloves should be recommended.
● Topical applications that may be tried are:
  –Emollients
  –Topical corticosteroids
  –Tar preparations.

17

Treatment of itch

BACKGROUND

It is sad that there is no surefire way of suppressing the common and often disabling symptom of pruritus. The act of scratching may evoke sniggers and mild amusement in onlookers but when persistent the symptom is anything but funny. It causes sleeplessness and eventually exhaustion and depression. Clearly the most satisfactory treatment of itch would be to remove its cause but in many patients the cause is obscure or irremediable. The first priority, then, is to reach a conclusion concerning the diagnosis by physical examination and laboratory investigation if required.

DIAGNOSIS

Itch caused by skin disease

Localized itch is more often due to an identifiable skin disorder than generalized itch. Pubic lice are occasionally the cause of itch around the genitalia and over the lower abdomen. Always inspect the area very carefully for nits or crab lice. Generalized atopic dermatitis is probably the commonest cause of severe itchiness but, less commonly, thick patches of dermatitis (circumscribed neurodermatitis or lichen simplex chronicus) may cause intense irritation at the back of the scalp, or near the elbows, wrists or ankles, and is usually easily identifiable. The elderly often have generalized irritation associated with their dry skin. This is made worse by an environment starved of humidity by central heating, or by frequent hot baths. Lichen planus can also produce unpleasant itch; this condition can be either localized or generalized. Psoriasis is not generally an itchy disorder but it may cause the symptom on the scalp or in the flexures.

Some men have intense itchiness around the anus (pruritus ani) which seems to persist unremittingly for many years. Persistent irritation of the same type is found in women but tends to be more perigenital. Despite sympathy, investigation, treatment and reassurance it is rare to find causes to account for the symptom in this group of patients; they remain a mystery and a problem in management (see Chapter 8).

Detailed inspection of the wrists, buttocks, genitalia and soles of the feet, in a good light and with a magnifying glass if necessary, will reveal scabies in a few patients – and save later embarrassment. A young woman complained to me of generalized itchiness for the previous six weeks. There were no particular clues in the story she told,

---

Some skin diseases that can cause itch

● Atopic dermatitis
● Dry skin of the elderly
● Other forms of dermatitis
● Scabies
● Ringworm
● Lichen simplex chronicus
● Pubic lice
● Psoriasis of the scalp
● Flexural psoriasis
● Candidiasis
● Lichen planus
● Dermatitis herpetiformis

---

and a cursory physical examination revealed no abnormality. A close look on the soles of feet, however, revealed two typical scabies runs and a mite nestling at the end of one of them.

Itch caused by systemic disease

If there is no obvious skin disorder responsible for the symptom then the possibility of underlying serious systemic disease has to be borne in mind as a cause. Obstructive jaundice, severe renal disease, thyroid disease disorders of calcium balance, Hodgkin's disease and blood dyscrasias occasionally cause pruritus and appropriate investigations should be initiated to exclude these possibilities. Diabetes is sometimes given as a cause of generalized itch but I have never seen a patient present in this way. However, diabetes can cause local perianal or perigenital itch from the candidiasis to which these patients are prone.

Nondisease

When examination fails to reveal any skin disease and systemic investigation reveals no abnormality, and the patient still complains bitterly of continued itchiness, all one's physicianly skills are required. It is not reasonable to transfer the blame to the patient

---

Some systemic diseases that can cause itch

● Obstructive jaundice
● Severe renal disease
● Disorders of calcium balance
● Hodgkin's disease and other lymphomatous disorders
● Blood dyscrasias

---

by labelling him or her 'neurotic'. Nonetheless it has to be said that there is a group of patients with generalized itch (mostly middle-aged women) in whom the only finding is the presence of scratch marks and small scratched papules (prurigo papules). The cause of this condition is unknown but could be primarily psychological in origin (see Chapter 8).

MANAGEMENT

The symptom of itchiness is usually worse at night in bed when the patient is warm and bedclothes are in contact with the skin. Light, smooth bedclothes are best and efforts should be made to stay cool.

Hot baths frequently bring on attacks of intolerable itching in some patients. Showering or bathing in tepid water with gentle patting dry afterwards should prevent this.

Woolly or other types of fluffy or abrasive clothing can exacerbate itching and atopics often find such clothing quite unwearable. Fine cotton and synthetic fabrics are better for these patients.

TREATMENT

Topical applications

Treatment of any underlying skin disorder is mandatory, but when none can be identified the simplest of topical remedies should be tried first.

Emollients Emollient soaps (such as unguentum emulsificans BP or E45 wash cream) and simple emollient creams or lotions usually provide some relief. Bathing (in warm, *not* hot water) with bath additives, such as oils (Oilatum emollient or Balneum) or oatmeal preparations, can give relief to some patients. Calamine lotion BPC is sometimes useful for localized itchy areas, but I prefer oily calamine lotion (calamine liniment) as this does not dry to a powder. The inclusion of ¼ or ½ per cent menthol may give greater relief at times.

Tars These seem to exert a mild antipruritic effect in some disorders. Preparations containing tar give some relief in dermatitic conditions – particularly chronic localized patches.

Local anaesthetic preparations Some of these preparations, such as those containing procaine, amethocaine or cinchocaine, give temporary relief from pruritus ani or pruritus vulvae but unfortunately there is an appreciable risk of sensitization with the latter two and allergic contact dermatitis. Preparations containing procaine are available in pharmacies and are much less likely to cause sensitization.

Antihistamine creams These are also used to relieve local itches – especially from insect bites – but are not very efficient. They are also capable of causing allergic contact dermatitis.

Systemic treatments

Systemic treatments for itchiness are not very effective.

Antihistamines Older antihistamines, such as chlorpheniramine (Piriton) and promethazine (Phenergan), give very little relief from itch except in some patients with urticaria. Their major action in other itchy states is to cause some drowsiness and sedation. Newer drugs, including terfenadine (Triludan), astemizole (Hismanal) and loratadine (Clarityn) are effective antihistamines. They do not cause drowsiness and do not relieve itch that is not due to urticaria.

Aspirin This can give relief from pruritus to some patients and this simple remedy is worth a trial. Topical corticosteroids only give relief from pruritus if the itching is caused by some inflammatory disorder, such as dermatitis. They have no intrinsic antipruritic activity.

PRACTICAL POINTS

- In many patients who present with itch as the only symptom the cause is obscure.
- Accurate diagnosis, even if only of nondisease, is essential before the problem can be tackled.
- Localized itch is more likely to result from a specific skin disease than generalized itch.
- Patients with itch should be advised:
  –To keep cool at night
  –To avoid taking hot baths
  –To avoid woollen clothing.
- Topical treatment is usually more successful than systemic.
- Simple preparations, such as emollients and tars, may be all that are needed for the relief of itch.

18

Treatment of dry skin

BACKGROUND

There are many disorders in which scaling and roughness of the skin surface are the predominant abnormalities. At one end of the scale this is a trivial problem verging on a question of aesthetics, while at the other end there are patients who are virtually crippled by gross scaling, thickening of the skin surface and consequent fissuring. The disorders which qualify for inclusion in this group include the congenital disorders of keratinization, the dry skin of the elderly (see Chapter 7) and atopic dermatitis (see Chapter 15). Of course the way that the scaling develops in each of these diseases differs and it must be appreciated that dry skin is a physical sign and not a disease in itself. It is only because there are no specific treatments for the underlying diseases that one is driven to use symptomatic treatments. For reasons not currently understood, not all body areas are affected equally. The extensor areas are worst affected and the shins and outer aspects of the upper arms seem particularly badly hit.

Although 'dry skin' seems an appropriate term for these conditions, the dryness is an illusion. We associate the irregular spikiness to the touch and the unevenness to the eye with dry physical objects. In addition, when the abnormal skin surface is hydrated it is immediately improved and this seems to confirm that the scaling and irregularity is due to a deficiency of water. In fact in some disorders the superficial scales may well contain more water than normal, rather than less. In any event the addition of water via one or other mechanism does improve the appearance and feel of the skin and provides temporary relief from the itchiness and soreness associated with the scaling.

The major causes of scaling

- Eczema – all varieties
- Skin infections, eg, ringworm
- Psoriasis
- Other inflammatory disorders of the skin
- Ichthyotic disorders and other congenital disorders of keratinization

---

Paradoxically, frequent immersion in water does not hydrate the skin but seems to make the scaling condition worse! It seems that the frequent addition of moisture and subsequent drying leaches out materials which are in some way vital to the horny layer. Finally this process of hydration and dehydration leads to chapping, fissuring, inflammation and eventually dermatitis.

TREATMENTS

Emollients

Emollients hydrate the skin surface by producing an oily occlusive film on the surface which allows a build-up of moisture from the epidermis. They are usually emulsions of some sort but modern pharmaceutical manipulation has created a wide variety of creaminess. The best emollient is one which the patient uses because he or she finds that it helps and is cosmetically acceptable. The beneficial effects of emollients start to wear off after three or four hours and one disadvantage of using them is that they need to be applied more than twice daily for the best result.

There are other ways of obtaining an emollient effect. Bath oils (Oilatum emollient, for example) may help by leaving a thin film of oil on the skin surface after bathing. Similarly, washing materials that have the cleansing effect of soap without actually containing soap are occasionally helpful (eg, emulsifying ointments BP, Oilatum soap, Neutrogena soap).

Keratolytics

Agents that promote desquamation (keratolytics) smooth the skin surface and are also used in the treatment of scaling dry skin conditions. Salicylic acid in concentrations of 1–6 per cent is used for this purpose. Urea, lactic acid and pyrrolidone carboxylic acid are supposed to have particular effects in assisting the stratum corneum to retain water and are sometimes included in emollients. They are known as humectants.

PRACTICAL ADVICE

Apart from applications of this or that emollient and special washing materials, practical everyday advice is important for dry-skinned patients. They should be told that centrally heated environments make their condition worse and that if they have central heating at home they should take care that there is also some humidification mechanism. A simple way of doing this is by placing dishes of water on the radiators.

Frequent hot baths are bad for dry skin. When sufferers do bathe or shower it should be in tepid water and with a soap substitute of some kind (see above). Patting dry is better than vigorous towelling.

Most people with dry itchy skin cannot tolerate wool or other fuzzy materials that come into contact with the skin and they should be advised to wear cotton or synthetic fabrics next to the skin.

PRACTICAL POINTS

● Disorders associated with chronically dry skin include:
–Congenital disorders of keratinization
–Dry skin of the elderly
–Atopic dermatitis
–Wasting diseases.
● Although the addition of water initially improves the skin's appearance and helps reduce itch, frequent immersion worsens the condition.
● Topical treatments for dry skin include:
–Emollients
–Keratolytics.
● Patients should be advised:
–To ensure that their home environment is humidified if centrally heated
–To take tepid showers rather than hot baths
–To avoid woolly clothing.

19
Treatment of psoriasis

BACKGROUND

As is probably appreciated by the reader, psoriasis is a persistent and recurrent inflammatory skin disease for which there is currently no long-term cure. However, there are ways of inducing remissions or at least improving virtually all patients with the disorder. In this chapter I shall be discussing treatments suitable for patients with mild or moderate psoriasis, as well as some of the effects of treatments given for patients with the more severe forms of the disease, which are commenced by specialist departments and may be continued as out-patient therapy in the community.

REASSURANCE AND ENCOURAGEMENT

Nothing is more depressing to a patient with psoriasis than to be told that it is incurable. Many patients with psoriasis have arrived at my clinic or been brought there by a relative in a depressed and agitated state. They had been told by someone along the line that there was little that could be done for them. Apart from the tremendous harm this must do to an individual's confidence and sense of well-being, it is just not true. As stated above, the great majority of patients can be cleared of the rash or at least considerably improved. All patients will require some explanation of the nature of the disorder and if thought appropriate they should be encouraged to join a recognized self-help group (see the list of useful addresses at the end of this book).

TOPICAL TREATMENTS

White soft paraffin

When there are just a few plaques, very little more than the rubbing in of white soft paraffin (Vaseline) once or twice a day need be recommended. Other emollients may be tried – in general, the thicker and greasier they are the more effective they are. The least they will do is to improve the appearance and decrease the scaling.

If there are one or two thickly encrusted patches then it is sometimes useful to apply a salicylic acid preparation for a week or two to remove the scale. Two to six per cent salicylic acid in white soft paraffin is useful for this purpose.

Tars

If further treatment is required a tar preparation can be prescribed. Tar ointment is the simplest but not the most elegant cosmetically. There are several quite good proprietary preparations, such as Clinitar or Alphosyl.

For psoriasis of the groin, navel and the submammary areas a weak tar cream (eg, Alphosyl) can be tried although even this is often irritating. For this type of psoriasis topical corticosteroids may be better (see opposite).

Unfortunately some tar preparations tend to be messy and may stain. Patients should be warned of this and told to use only a thin smear, as well as to cover the treated sites with cotton gauze or some other type of light dressing. Tar can also cause redness and soreness on sun exposed areas ('tar smarts') and may also cause an acne type of folliculitis in some patients.

Dithranol

If tars are ineffective then use can be made of the proprietary preparations of dithranol (eg, Dithrocream, Dithrolan, Exolan, Psoradate and Stie–Lasan). At one time dithranol treatment was almost totally restricted to in-patients. This need no longer be the case. Nonetheless the preparations available are not perfect and still produce characteristic staining of the skin, clothes and bedclothes. They also tend to irritate the skin and the patient must be warned of this possibility. Both tar and dithranol preparations need only

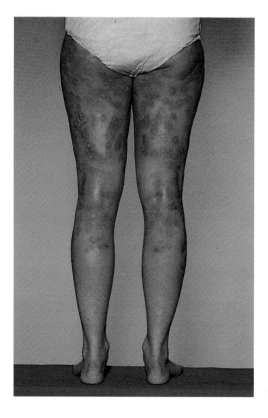

Typical mauvish-brown staining from dithranol treatment.

be applied once daily in most patients. More frequent applications rarely give added benefit. Tar and dithranol applications take at least three weeks to produce improvement but it can be as long as eight weeks before improvement is obvious.

Calcipotriol

Calcipotriol (Donovex) is an analogue of vitamin D that, when used in a concentration of 50 µg/g, has been found to be very effective for plaque-type psoriasis. It may be expected to clear or considerably improve psoriatic lesions in approximately 65 per cent of patients in an eight to ten week period. Its only major disadvantage is a propensity to irritate the skin – preventing its use by 20 to 25 per cent of subjects. Other vitamin D analogues are being developed and will be available in the near future.

Corticosteroids

There was a vogue for the use of potent topical corticosteroids in psoriasis. There is little doubt that they can rapidly improve the lesions but unfortunately the disadvantages of their use in this disease outweigh their advantages. It seems that in most psoriatic patients the suppression of the disease that the topical corticosteroids induce is operative only while the preparation is being used. Immediately it is stopped the disease tends to return. What is more, it sometimes seems to return with additional vigour. In addition, these compounds may have unpleasant side-effects both locally and systemically as a result of absorption (see Chapter 27).

It would be misleading to suggest that there is absolutely no place for the use of topical corticosteroids in psoriasis, but many dermatologists would agree that they have a very limited role to play. Corticosteroid creams or lotions can, however, be very useful for

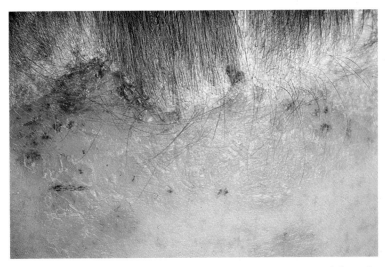

The scalp margin of a man with psoriasis. Note the thick crusting of the scalp skin. Frequent regular shampooing with a tar-based shampoo as well as application of an appropriate topical preparation is the best treatment.

psoriasis of the groin, the navel and the submammary areas. If they are used for this type of psoriasis it is important to make sure that the condition being treated is in fact psoriasis and not ringworm or thrush. They are also sometimes useful in psoriasis of the scalp and flexures of the face.

Shampoos

Psoriasis of the scalp can be difficult to treat. It is best to advise that the patient adopt a short hair style to allow frequent shampooing. When the scalp is quite thickly encrusted it should be shampooed on alternate days at least and preferably every day. A regimen I often recommend is application of an ointment at night and shampooing first thing in the morning. This leaves the scalp free of messy ointments during the day. As far as the actual shampoos and applications are concerned, a tar-based shampoo (eg, Polytar liquid) and a tar-and-salicylic acid ointment is quite useful. If this doesn't do the trick then a weak or moderately potent corticosteroid cream can be applied after shampooing.

For psoriasis of the nails

Unfortunately there is no effective topical remedy for psoriasis of the nails. When the nail involvement is not severe, all that needs to be done is to keep the nails short. Injection of corticosteroid suspensions around the nail beds has been tried but is painful and not very effective. If there is severe nail involvement then this will be a factor in persuading the specialist that systemic therapy is indicated.

SYSTEMIC TREATMENTS

After discharge from hospital a patient with severe psoriasis may still be receiving treatment with methotrexate, etretinate (Tigason) or PUVA and it is important to mention some of the questions that the practitioner may have in relation to these.

Treatments for psoriasis

Topical
- White soft paraffin (Vaseline) with or without salicylic acid
- Tars
- Dithranol preparations
- Calcipotriol
- Corticosteroids
- Tar-based shampoos

Systemic
- Methotrexate
- Etretinate (Tigason)
- Cyclosporin
- Photochemotherapy with ultraviolet type A (PUVA)

Methotrexate

Methotrexate treatment is usually given by mouth once weekly, although in some patients it is given by injection. It must be taken regularly to maintain its effect. Alcoholic drinks should be drastically reduced or prohibited during methotrexate treatment as severe liver damage is a not infrequent result of the combination. It can cause indigestion, nausea and vague abdominal discomforts. More serious side-effects to look out for include agranulocytosis, liver damage and susceptibility to infection. If other drugs have to be given during methotrexate treatment, enquiry should be made as to their interaction with methotrexate. Particular care should be taken with salicylates and other antirheumatics as they may interfere with the excretion of methotrexate. This may be a particular problem in the elderly who may already have a compromised renal function. Pregnancy must be avoided while on this drug as it is teratogenic. A total cumulative dose of >1.5 g of methotrexate has been associated with hepatocellular damage and fibrosis. Particular caution is needed in patients who have taken the drug for more than one year. Some advocate liver biopsy after six months of treatment.

Etretinate

Etretinate (Tigason) is given daily by mouth and usually takes some four to six weeks before it starts to work. It does not usually give rise to intestinal symptoms but nearly always causes dryness and cracking of the lips. Some slight and temporary increased rate of loss of scalp hair may occur while on the drug. Other problems that occasionally occur with etretinate include dryness and itchiness of the skin, stickiness of the skin and nose bleeds. The drug can also cause hyperlipidaemia in some 25 per cent of patients and this should be checked by blood tests. In some patients who are on etretinate for longer periods and on high dosage, ossification may occur in ligaments and interosseous membranes. The disseminated interstitial skeletal hyperostosis syndrome may be seen in patients on long-term treatment but does not seem to compromise mobility in the large majority of patients. Etretinate is teratogenic and effective contraception must be used both while on the drug and for two years afterwards as it persists in the body for very long periods.

Acitretin (Neotigason), which is very similar to etretinate, has been introduced recently. It is more water soluble than etretinate and has slightly different pharmacokinetics – only 70 per cent of the dose of etretinate is required. Its efficacy and side-effect profile are exactly the same as for etretinate. Unfortunately a small proportion is actually metabolized to etretinate and therefore the implications with regard to teratogenicity are the same. In the United Kingdom, acitretin has supplemented etretinate and is only available from hospital pharmacies.

PUVA

PUVA (photochemotherapy with A-type ultraviolet radiation) has been in use in some hospitals and special clinics since the mid-1970s. Patients take a psoralen (8-methoxypsoralen or 5-methoxypsoralen) and receive UVA irradiation from special lamps some two hours later. Treatment is usually given three or four times per week at first but may be needed only once or twice a week during maintenance therapy. Patients receiving PUVA become quite tanned. This fact plus the lack of messy ointments makes this treatment popular with many patients.

Some psoriatics feel claustrophobic in PUVA cabinets and some larger patients cannot actually fit into them. These drawbacks and the occasional sunburn from overenthusiastic treatment apart, the treatment is remarkably trouble-free in the short term. There is some concern about carcinogenic effects on the skin in the long term, and fair-skinned subjects who are susceptible to the effects of sunlight are generally not considered for treatment. At the time of writing it is acknowledged that there is a much higher incidence of squamous cell carcinoma in patients who have received many PUVA treatments.

PRACTICAL POINTS

- Although there is no cure for psoriasis, patients should be reassured that much can be done to clear their rash or at least to greatly alleviate their condition.
- White soft paraffin, with 2–6 per cent salicylic acid if necessary, is indicated for mild psoriasis.
- Tars and dithranol should be prescribed for more extensive and persistent scaling plaques of psoriasis.
- Tar-based shampoos and tar-and-salicylic-acid ointments are the first-line treatments for psoriasis of the scalp.
- Calcipotriol is a useful topical treatment for plaque-type psoriasis.
- Topical corticosteroids should not usually be prescribed for psoriasis except when it occurs in the groin, the navel or the submammary areas, and occasionally for psoriasis of the scalp.
- Systemic treatments are for severe cases only and should be commenced by specialists.

20

Treatment of exudative rashes and conditions that blister

EXUDATIVE RASHES

Localized

Dermatitis can begin with startling ferocity. When it does, the affected area becomes red and swollen and exudes a serous fluid. Psoriasis can also be quite inflamed, although usually less markedly so than with dermatitis. It doesn't exude in the same way but pustules may appear over the affected surface. Erysipelas can appear on the face or leg quite dramatically. The involved area is red, swollen and very tender. Other localized skin infections can also start suddenly and require urgent treatment.

Treatment These sorts of acute rashes should be treated gently. Exuding areas can be bathed with saline compresses or a mild astringent such as very dilute potassium permanganate (1:8000). It is also advisable to keep the patient (and the affected part) at rest as much as possible.

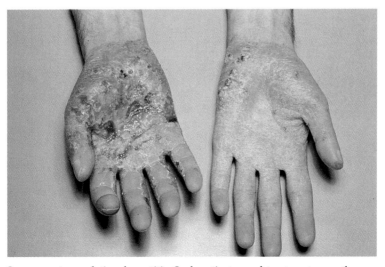

Severe, acute exudative dermatitis. Such patients need treatment urgently.

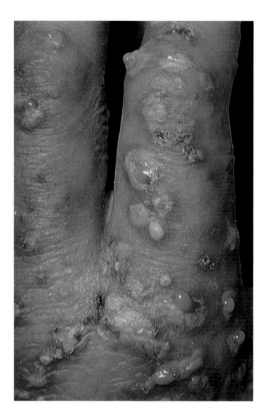

Severe infected dermatitis. Notice the many pustules containing yellowish pus. This patient needs urgent treatment with antibiotics after swabs have been taken for culture.

Sedation and analgesia may be required as this type of violent eruption is disturbing and can be painful. Antibiotics will also be required if the lesions become infected.

Widespread

Several skin disorders can suddenly become generalized (erythrodermic), including psoriasis, dermatitis and drug-induced eruptions (see Chapter 13). When an appreciable proportion of the skin surface is involved in this way there are general points in management to be remembered, apart from just treatment of the rash itself (see above).

1. Heat loss from large areas of inflamed skin may be considerable and the sufferer may complain of feeling cold and may actually shiver. Such patients should be kept warm to avoid the danger of hypothermia.
2. Blood flow to the inflamed skin is greatly increased and this acts as a 'peripheral shunt' which results in increased cardiac stroke volume and cardiac output. People with young and healthy hearts can withstand this quite well, but the elderly may just be tipped into cardiac failure by the increased load on the myocardium.
3. Dehydration occurs very quickly because of the increased water loss across the damaged skin and some patients complain of feeling thirsty.

Causes of erythroderma

- Psoriasis
- Dermatitic eruptions – particularly severe atopic dermatitis and seborrhoeic dermatitis in elderly
- Drug eruptions (eg, hydantoinates, antirheumatic drugs)
- Reticuloses affecting the skin – mycosis fungoides
- Pityriasis rubra pilaris
- Rare forms of ichthyosis
- Unknown causes

Complications of erythroderma

Complications	Possible effects
Disturbances of heat balance due to loss of heat from skin	– May lead to hypothermia
Disturbances of fluid balance due to loss of stratum corneum barrier function	– May lead to dehydration
Disturbances of circulatory system due to increased blood flow through skin and inflamed skin capillaries	– May lead to hyperdynamic circulation and even heart failure; may cause oedema in some sites
Nutritional disturbances due to high metabolic rate of inflamed skin	– May cause functional disturbance of intestinal epithelium – 'dermatogenic enteropathy' and haematological disorders
General systemic disturbance	– May cause extreme malaise and depression

Luckily such extensive and inflamed rashes occur infrequently, but when they do occur it must be remembered that the whole patient is sick, not just the skin.

CONDITIONS THAT BLISTER

The sudden onset of widespread blistering is always disturbing. Although it may arise from a trivial and self-limiting cause, such as chickenpox or multiple insect bites, it may also announce the onset of a more threatening disease, such as pemphigus or pemphigoid (see Chapter 37).

Treatment

The affected individual needs to be observed carefully to determine whether early in-patient treatment will be required.

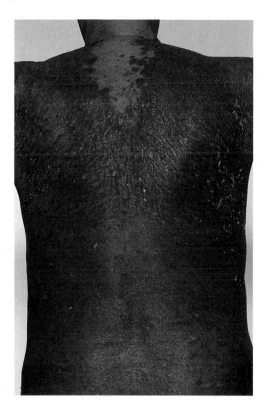

Erythrodermic psoriasis. This man had had typical psoriasis since childhood which occasionally became universally red as shown in this photograph of his back. The loss of heat and fluid from the skin dictates that efficient treatment is given early in the disease.

I am often asked whether blisters should be pricked with a needle to empty them. In general they should be left alone although if very large it may be kinder to prick them with a sterile needle. Blistered areas need to be kept clean and moist; wet, sterile, saline gauze compresses are suitable as an emergency measure.

BPRACTICAL POINTS

● Exudative rashes should be bathed gently with saline compresses or a mild astringent.
● Sedatives and analgesics may also be required.
● Widespread blistering may indicate serious disease.
● Blistering areas should be kept clean and moist.

21

Treatment of acne

BACKGROUND

Most people have acne spots to some degree at some time during adolescence and part of the skill in treating the disease is knowing which patients to treat and when. The following are general hints which should be helpful to the inexperienced practitioner:

1. What seems trivial acne to you may be of enormous concern to the young-ster in front of you and will probably require treatment.
2. The whole of the affected zone should be treated to prevent invisibly affected follicles being the focus of new lesions.
3. Acne spots that appear on the chin and return with each menstrual period are difficult to improve and it is probably more useful to attempt to modulate the menses rather than the skin.
4. At times it may be necessary to use both topical and systemic treatments.
5. The disease can be provoked by drugs (steroids or testosterone), by indus-trial exposure (chloracne from dioxin absorption, or exposure of skin to cutting oils for instance) and by application of oils and greases to the skin. The correct approach in these situations is to remove the initiating or aggra-vating factor.

The following general advice may be helpful to patients:

1. There is no evidence that acne is caused or made worse by what one eats or drinks, neither has it been shown that acne can be improved by altering the diet.
2. Acne is not due to uncleanliness or lack of washing, so there is little point in getting patients to scrub their skins thoroughly until raw. Normal washing is sufficient.
3. There is no evidence that too much (or too little) sexual activity has any causative or provocative role in acne and no special advice on this aspect of the patient's life need be given other than to behave as normal.
4. Some encouragement towards outdoor activities can be useful as gentle exposure to the sun does help some patients.
5. Many acne patients pick, push and pull their spots almost uncontrollably. Apart from tying their hands behind their backs there is little to be done as in most dermatologists' experience even stern advice does little to curb their

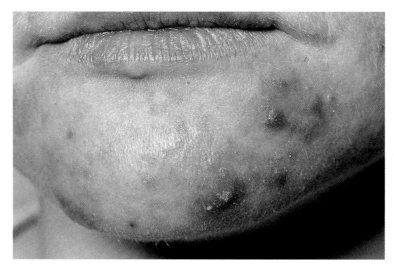

Acne affecting the chin and lower face in a young woman.

compulsive fiddling. Nonetheless it should be explained that continual picking at the lesions does tend to make the scars more noticeable.
6. Cosmetics should be permitted – provided they are not too heavy or greasy (see Chapter 10). It is the heavier foundations that can make the condition worse.

All patients with acne can be helped by treatment, although it may need to be continued for long periods. If there appears to be little improvement it is probably best to refer the patient for specialist advice.

TOPICAL TREATMENTS

These are suitable for most acne patients except perhaps in cases where vast expanses of the body are covered with deep lesions. The available treatments are designed either to increase the rate of desquamation of surface scale from the skin and so get rid of blackheads, or to reduce the numbers of skin bacteria. A few topical agents used in acne may act via an anti-inflammatory effect. A detailed description of all available lotions, gels and creams would require a book in itself; a few general comments will suffice here.

Antiseptic washes (eg, pHiso-MED) do little harm and may do some good. There is some argument as to the usefulness of applications that contain sulphur. I think that 3–5 per cent sulphur in calamine lotion or some other vehicle can deal with mild superficial acne. Benzoyl peroxide-containing applications in 5 or 10 per cent concentrations (eg, Panoxyl) are probably the most effective topical agents. They are available as lotions, creams or gels. Some preparations of benzoyl peroxide include other agents (eg, an antimicrobial as in Benzamycin and Quinoderm).

Tretinoin as 0.01 or 0.025 per cent lotion, gel or cream (Retin-A) is quite helpful to some patients. Topical isotretinoin (Isotrex) is also useful. Both these topical retinoids are

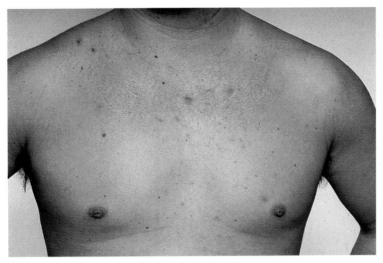

An irritant reaction of the skin due to use of a 5 per cent benzoyl peroxide-
containing gel used for the treatment of acne. Notice that the skin is pink and
shows some slight scaling and fissuring in places.

especially helpful for patients with superficial acne characterized by many comedones
and pustules. New topical retinoids are likely to be available in the next few years.
Azelaic acid (Skinoren) has antimicrobial effects and probably helps remove comedones
too. It is nonirritating and helps patients with milder types of acne.

Unfortunately all these applications can irritate the skin if used too frequently, and some
sufferers, particularly those with fair skin, seem quite unable to tolerate certain preparations.

Topical antibiotics are quite popular, clean and nonirritating acne treatments: tetracycline (eg, Topicycline), clindamycin (Dalacin T) and erythromycin (eg, Stiemycin and
Zineryt). These agents are among the most effective topical anti-acne treatments.

SYSTEMIC TREATMENTS

Orally administered antibiotics are the mainstay of treatment for moderately severe or
severe acne. Tetracycline (or another member of the tetracycline group) and erythromycin
are the ones that are generally used and appear most helpful. Treatment should start with
250 mg given three times or twice per day and continued at that dose until improvement
begins. This usually happens after some six to ten weeks but in some cases may take four
or five months. Treatment with antibiotics may need to be continued for one or two years.

Treatment with the retinoid drug isotretinoin (Roaccutane) has proved dramatically
successful for many patients with severe and cystic acne. Isotretinoin is the most effective of systemic treatments for severe acne. It is usually given for a 4 month course
in the first instance, at a dose of 1 mg/kg/day; this regimen clears some 70–80 per
cent of patients. It seems to work mainly by cutting down sebum secretion. As with
the other retinoid drugs given systemically – etretinate and acitretin – isotretinoin is
only available from hospital pharmacies. Side-effects are similar to those caused by

etretinate (see page 121) and include dry lips, drying of other mucosae, transient increase in loss of scalp hair, increase in blood lipids, hepatic damage and bony problems. Teratogenicity is also a serious risk and all women in the reproductive age group must take effective contraceptive measures while taking the drug and for two months after stopping.

The combination of an anti-androgen – cyproterone acetate – and an oestrogen – ethinyloestradiol, known as Dianette – is an effective hormonal anti-acne treatment for young women. It suppresses ovulation and acts as an oral contraceptive.

SURGERY

There is little place for surgery in draining cystic lesions, as bad hypertrophic or keloid scars often result. If large cysts need to be drained the contents can be aspirated through a large-bore needle and a corticosteroid suspension instilled afterwards.

Dermabrasion has been used to help the superficial pit and pock scars that disturb some patients. This measure can improve the appearance in fair-skinned patients but darker subjects may end up with an odd mottled pigmentation.

Frequently prescribed treatments for acne

Topical
- Antiseptic washes
- Topical antimicrobial agents
- Sulphur in calamine lotion
- Benzoyl peroxide applications
- Tretinoin or isotretinoin lotions, gels and creams
- Topical antibiotics
- Topical azelaic acid

Systemic
- Antibiotics
  –Tetracycline group
  –Erythromycin
- Isotretinoin (specialist use only)
- Cyproterone acetate and ethinyloestradiol

PRACTICAL POINTS

- There is no evidence that acne is related to diet, cleanliness or sexual activity.
- Gentle exposure to the sun often helps.
- All patients can be helped by treatment:
  –Topical treatments are effective for most patients
  –Systemic treatments can be used for more severe cases.

22

When and how to treat viral warts

BACKGROUND

Viral warts can become a major nuisance for practitioners and it is a good idea to develop a treatment policy towards them.

First, make sure that what are presented as warts are in fact viral warts. Beware of the solitary wart in the elderly as squamous cell carcinoma can present as a solitary warty nodule. They can also be confused with solar keratoses or seborrhoeic warts (see Chapters 7 and 36).

Perianal or genital warts in the sexually active age groups may be what they seem but may also be a manifestation of secondary syphilis (condyloma lata). The heaped and slightly warty lesions of secondary syphilis are usually soggier and more prolific than ordinary genital warts. In addition there are usually other signs of syphilis present.

In children or young adults, wart-like lesions that are small, dome-shaped, whitish papules with a central warty spot are probably the lesions of another virus infection – molluscum contagiosum.

In most cases warts resolve spontaneously, so that whatever you do may appear effective. Unfortunately their resolution is unpredictable and some warts seem to take forever to disappear. The old wives' tales of warts vanishing after they have been bought for a penny or after burying a steak in the garden or after some other equally bizarre magical technique are (at least partially) explicable on the basis of this tendency to spontaneous regression. However, practitioners should try especially hard to clear some warts before natural resolution in certain situations.

PLANTAR WARTS

Warts on the soles of the feet tend to develop callosities over them and become painful. These should be pared down carefully or scraped with a pumice stone and a salicylic acid preparation applied. Collodion flex containing salicylic acid is suitable, as are combinations of salicylic and lactic acid (Salactol, Compound W), or one of the proprietary salicylic acid plasters can be used. The treated area should be covered with an occlusive plaster. When effective the wart turns white and the area becomes slightly tender. If this is ineffective then a podophyllin preparation can be employed. Podophyllin is a mixture of toxic alkaloids obtained by extracting the root of the

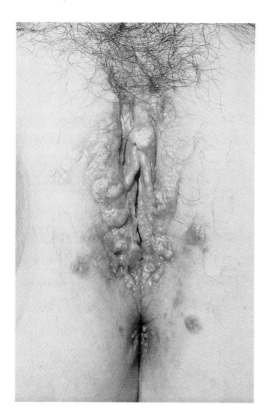

Condylomata lata (lesions of secondary syphilis) around the vulva of a young woman. Her serological tests for syphilis were positive.

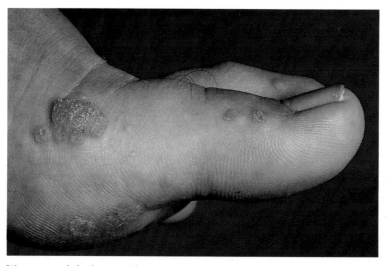

Warts around the big toe. Plantar warts can be very painful.

mandrake plant. There are podophyllin paints and collodion flex preparations as well as proprietary ointment preparations (Posalfilin). The latter are particularly useful for plantar warts; the paints and flexes are more useful for genital warts (see opposite). Treatment with formalin or glutaraldehyde had a vogue but does not seem to have much advantage over other treatments.

If these measures do not work then locally destructive treatment by freezing with liquid nitrogen or a cryoprobe, or electrocautery and curettage, will be required. These methods of treatment are usually available in hospital out-patient clinics but the waiting lists for patients with warts are often so long that the warts resolve before the appointment comes round. Even these vigorous procedures do not always succeed and warts often recur at the treated sites. If treatment is too vigorous, permanently painful scars can result, for which no one is thanked.

MULTIPLE WARTS

Solitary warts on the hands or two or three on the fingers don't often need treatment but when there are multiple warts on the fingers and around the nails (paronychial) active treatment should be considered. The same treatments are available for these as for plantar warts, and they are generally more successful for these lesions.

Plane warts on the face, neck or hands don't often need treatment, but if multiple lesions are present then one of the liquid salicylic acid or salicylic-lactic acid film preparations (such as Duofilm) is suitable.

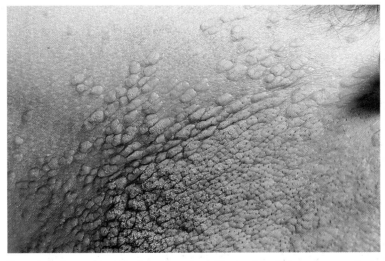

Extensive plane warts affecting the neck and lower face. This young man had suffered from these for many years. There was no identified immune defect in this patient.

GENITAL AND PERIANAL WARTS

These always need treatment as they tend to spread quickly to sexual partners (Chapter 9). Tincture of podophyllin is the most popular treatment for these and is best carried out by a specialist department. Usually treatment starts with a single application of a 5 per cent podophyllin solution which is washed off after four or five hours. If this is ineffective, stronger tinctures (up to 20 per cent) are used. In recent years the active alkaloid (podophyllotoxin) has been extracted from the resin and made available in a pure form as a 0.5 per cent paint (Condyline). If podophyllin treatment is successful, the warts become inflamed and painful and then drop off.

If podophyllin is unsuccessful then more vigorous destructive measures may be necessary, such as electrocautery. For obvious reasons this should be administered by an expert in this technique.

Perianal warts seem to be more common in male homosexuals, who are also prone to harbour other venereal disorders including HIV disease. It has become routine practice to check whether such patients have evidence of syphilis with blood tests.

PRACTICAL POINTS

- Viral warts may be confused with:
  –Seborrhoeic warts
  –Condyloma lata of syphilis
  –Molluscum contagiosum
  –Solar keratoses or squamous cell carcinoma.
- Most warts clear spontaneously.
- Be careful not to cause more discomfort with the treatment than the warts cause themselves.
- The following may require treatment:
  –Plantar warts
  –Multiple warts
  –Facial warts
  –Genital warts.
- First-line treatment for plantar warts is a salicylic acid preparation.
- First-line treatment for genital warts is a podophyllin preparation.

23
Treatment of leg ulcers

BACKGROUND

Chronic leg ulcers are a major cause of pain and discomfort and an economic burden on the community. They rarely attract the interest of doctors and there has been little advance in their management in recent years. It is important that some understanding of their nature and the way they respond to treatment is diffused into the medical community.

DIAGNOSIS

Gravitational ulcers

Persistent venous incompetence is by far and away the commonest reason for chronic ulceration of the lower legs. Gravitational ulcers tend to occur in the elderly at the lower end of the socioeconomic scale and ischaemia, nutritional deficiency and concomitant disease tend to be contributing causes.

Gravitational ulcers tend to have a slough-filled base, an irregular, slightly raised edge and pigmented, oedematous surrounding skin. They mostly occur just above the medial malleolus.

However, venous incompetence is not the only cause and to provide the ulcer sufferer with the proper treatment it is vital that the underlying reason for the complaint is identified.

Arterial ischaemia

The other major cause of leg ulceration is arterial ischaemia. These ulcers tend to be painful compared to gravitational ulcers, which in general give rise to less discomfort. They usually have sharply defined margins with surrounding skin that is shiny, hairless and atrophic. Ischaemic lesions may occur anywhere on the feet or ankles. They sometimes occur on the toes, dorsum or heel but can also occur around the malleoli.

Diabetes

People with diabetes are prone to leg ulcers of both the gravitational and arterial varieties. In addition, if they have neural involvement they may suffer from trophic ulceration at the sites of repeated trauma (the metatarsal arch, for example).

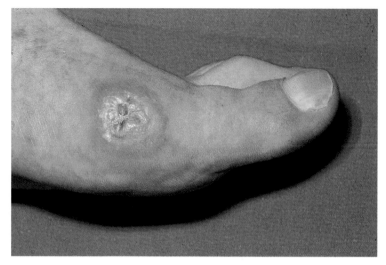

An ulcer due to peripheral arterial ischaemia. This was extremely painful and later the foot developed gangrenous changes.

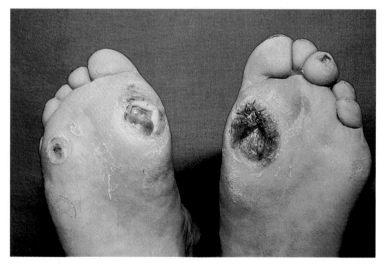

Severe neurotropic ulceration of the soles of a diabetic's feet. These ulcers often perforate (perforating ulcers) and are very disabling.

Blood disorders

It is wise to check for any haematological abnormality in a patient with a leg ulcer. Iron deficiency and normochromic normocytic anaemias occur in patients with long-standing ulceration. In addition sufferers from sickle cell disease, haemolytic diseases and platelet disorders may develop leg ulcers and their condition can be much improved if the disease is discovered and treated.

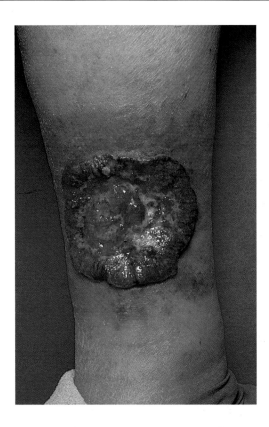

Squamous cell epithelioma of the lower leg. This lesion was treated for some time as a venous ulcer. The rolled and everted edge is typical of the neoplasm.

Vasculitis and pyoderma gangrenosum

When the walls of the small blood vessels are inflamed the term vasculitis is used. This can result in ischaemic necrosis of the skin involved, and ulceration. Rheumatoid arthritis is sometimes complicated by vasculitis of this sort and disabling persistent ulceration. The ulcers start off with blue-black swollen areas surrounded by a red flare. These break down and give rise to large ragged ulcers.

Pyoderma gangrenosum is fairly uncommon but rarely forgotten when seen for the first time. It is probably a type of vasculitis precipitated by underlying bowel disease, rheumatoid arthritis or gammopathy in some patients. The ulcer (or ulcers) can spread with alarming speed and reach quite frightening proportions. Such lesions are deep, and have an undermined edge and a raised bluish edge.

Other causes

There are many other causes of chronic ulcers, some rare, others not so rare, but the only ones that need to be mentioned here are the neoplastic group. It is only too easy to look at 'old Mr Brown's ulcer' over several years yet not actually see that it has enlarged and changed in character with a raised rolled edge. Squamous cell carcinoma and basal cell carcinoma can arise as a complication of persistent ulceration and also can start de novo in this area. To misdiagnose them is a major tragedy.

TREATMENT

Removal of the cause

Ideally, removal of the cause of the ulcer is the best treatment but regrettably this is rarely possible. Nonetheless, it is often possible to hasten healing by recognizing the nature of the underlying problem and taking steps to minimize the damage it causes or in some way counteract it. Here are two examples:

Gravitational ulceration Removal of the easily visible external varicose veins does little to alter the haemodynamics, and tying off perforating veins seems to help only occasionally. However, adequate support with well-applied elastic bandages or well-made stockings and regular rest with the leg elevated always gives some assistance.

Arterial ischaemia This can rarely be helped by simple measures and the drugs presently available to produce vasodilatation or to improve tissue nutrition in some other way rarely seem to do any good. If there is good evidence that the ulceration is due to major vessel disease the patient should be referred to a vascular surgeon for his opinion as to whether surgery will improve the situation.

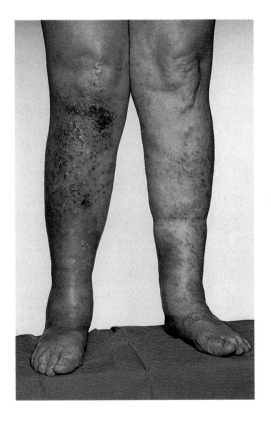

This patient with long-standing bilateral venous incompetence used an ointment containing neomycin and developed neomycin hypersensitivity to add to her problem.

Removal of slough, crust and clot

All other things being equal, ulcers can heal quite happily despite the presence of the most unpleasant slough and crust. Even so, this should be removed if it is offensive or appears to be impeding progress. If ordinary saline soaks don't seem to work, the enzyme preparation streptokinase/streptodornase (Varidase) can liquefy stubborn debris, and dextran polymer beads (Debrisan) can assist drainage of an ulcer with a slough-filled base. Benzoyl peroxide preparations, particularly a 20 per cent lotion (Benoxyl), are also useful in clearing up an ulcer and promoting the appearance of granulation tissue. An important ingredient of treatment is patience as tough adherent debris may take quite a time in separating.

Dressings and topical applications

Dressings should be performed daily or on alternate days depending on the amount of exudate. Ordinary moist saline gauze swabs are satisfactory providing that they remain damp – or else they adhere to the ulcer. Some nonadherent dressings such as paraffin-impregnated tulles are excellent, providing that they do not overhydrate the ulcer and surrounding skin or cause irritation of the ulcer. Hydrocolloid dressings and silicone

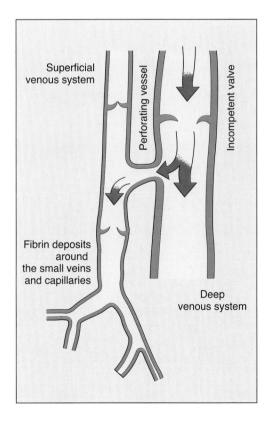

An incompetent valve in the deep venous system of the leg allows blood to flow backwards, increasing pressure in the superficial veins. This often leads to a build-up of fibrin deposits in and around the small intracutaneous and subcutaneous vessels.

foam dressings provide protection and hydration and seem free of toxic side-effects. These are certainly beneficial for some patients. There are some bandages that are impregnated with coal tar or other agents and are meant to stay in place for a week at a time or longer. My view is that they do little good and mainly serve only to put the problem out of sight.

Topical corticosteroids should not be used on ulcers; they slow down healing and encourage infection. Topical antibiotics serve little purpose and can also be harmful. Unfortunately at the time of writing there are no topical agents which actually promote healing; there are agents, however, that improve the 'local environment' and permit healing to occur.

Eczema may develop around gravitational ulcers. Often this is due to contact hyper-sensitivity to one of the medicaments. If this happens, the current topical applications should be stopped and something simple, such as zinc cream, should be applied pending investigation at a dermatology department.

Other measures

Patients should be encouraged to rest with their feet slightly elevated and to continue to take some exercise when not resting. Attention to coexistent medical problems is always important and special mention has already been made of the possible presence

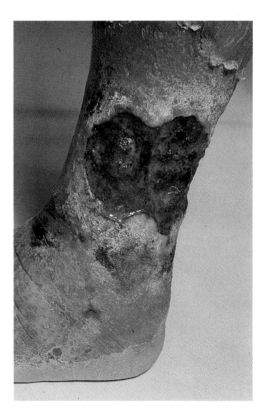

Typical gravitational ulcer. Despite treatment this lesion became infected. There is a greyish-green slough indicating an infection with Gram-negative bacteria. The ulcer had a copious foul-smelling discharge.

of anaemia. Most patients with gravitational ulcers are elderly and often socially deprived and may need the help of the available social agencies.

Patients with 'gravitational' syndrome have venous hypertension and seem to develop fibrin deposits in and around the small blood vessels in their legs. Attempts to counter-act this tendency have been made using fibrinolytic drugs – especially the anabolic agents, eg, stanozolol (Stromba).

INFECTION

Not surprisingly, ulcerated areas are easily colonized by all sorts of bacteria. Fortunately it is only rarely that extremely serious and life-threatening infection occurs. The surrounding skin becomes red and tender, the base of the ulcer becomes very exudative and the ulcer may begin to smell – particularly if Gram-negative bacteria are to blame. A pyrexia may develop and with some infections the patient may suddenly become very ill.

What to do?

In these cases treatment should be regarded as a matter of urgency. Swabs for bacterial culture and blood cultures should be taken, and immediately afterwards antibiotic treat-ment should be given. If hospital admission cannot be arranged quickly cephradine or ampicillin should be started.

Where minor degrees of infection are present that cause minimal symptoms and signs, topical treatments usually suffice. Removal of slough and exudate is achieved by bathing twice daily in dilute hydrogen peroxide solution or dilute potassium permanganate solution (1:8000). There is no place now for the old-fashioned vital dyes. These were pretty, but very damaging to the tissues. Topical antibiotics rarely possess the right spectrum of activities for all the infecting micro-organisms; they produce resistant strains and some can sensitize the surrounding skin and cause dermatitis. Povidone-iodine (Betadine) seems to possess none of these disadvantages and is a useful topical antibac-terial agent.

PRACTICAL POINTS

- Venous incompetence is the commonest cause of leg ulcers. Other causes include:
  −Arterial ischaemia
  −Loss of neural function, as in diabetes
  −Blood disorders
  −Neoplasia
  −Vasculitis.
- Elastic-bandage or stocking support and elevation of the affected leg help clear up ulcers due to venous incompetence. Fibrinolytic agents may help prevent ulceration.
- Stubborn slough or crust can be removed by bathing with saline or a weak antiseptic lotion or with streptokinase/streptodornase (Varidase) or dextran polymer beads (Debrisan).
- Dressings should be performed at least on alternate days.
- Cases of severe acute infection should be treated with appropriate antibiotics and may require cephradine or ampicillin straightaway if immediate hospital admission cannot be arranged.
- Minor ulcer infections may be treated topically with a peroxide or povidone-iodine preparation.

24

What can be done for hair loss and hirsutism?

HAIR LOSS

The cynical response to the first part of this question of 'not very much' is to be discouraged. An accurate diagnosis is the first necessity.

Male-pattern alopecia (androgenetic alopecia)

This is the commonest type of hair loss in men. It starts on the vertex and in either temple and gradually progresses to the classic bald pate. It is not associated with dandruff or any disease (or any sexual proclivity!).

At the time of writing, treatments to reverse or check the progress of male-pattern baldness are inadequate, inconvenient and not inexpensive. Transplantation of plugs of hair-bearing skin at the sides of the scalp to the bald areas certainly 'works'. Unfortunately unless the operator is experienced the scalp can end up looking like a 'shoe brush' with irregular tufts. The procedure is time-consuming and expensive but in

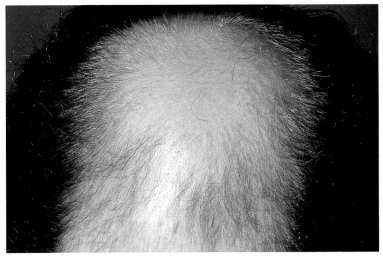

Typical male-pattern hair loss. The loss of hair from the temporal regions has progressed to join a similar deficient area over the vertex.

the right hands can produce good cosmetic results. Hair transplantation is much more often performed in the USA but is increasingly offered in Europe and elsewhere. 'Hair weaving' is safe but is expensive and gives an 'odd' look to the scalp. Implantation of nylon fibres can cause severe inflammation and scarring – it should be discouraged.

Apart from these surgical and cosmetic procedures I should also mention minoxidil as a pharmacological method of stimulating hair growth. Minoxidil (Regaine) lotion when used daily over some months will induce a minor degree of regrowth in up to 20–25 per cent of patients – but only for as long as it is used. It is safe but once again rather expensive to use.

For the majority of patients the most suitable treatment is explanation and reassurance. They should be warned off spending hard-earned money on quack remedies – of which there are many! Some 'self-conscious' men seem to benefit by wearing a toupee.

Hair loss in women

Diffuse hair loss in women is quite common and may be due to several different disorders. Most women lose some hair a few weeks to three months after childbirth. This is termed 'telogen defluvium' and is due to the systemic disturbance of childbirth which pushes many hair follicles into the resting or 'telogen' phase of the hair cycle. This is a normal physiological event and the hair subsequently regrows rapidly.

Male-pattern loss (better termed androgenetic alopecia) can also occur in women. It is not very common, but minor degrees are more frequent than generally thought. If severe and progressive, then specialist advice should be sought, because a masculinizing syndrome could be the cause. If this is the case there is usually also disturbance of the menstrual periods, and acne spots and seborrhoea may also occur.

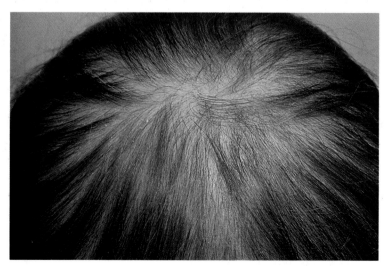

Telogen loss of hair in women sometimes occurs some weeks after delivery. The loss of hair can be quite extensive but recovers in a few weeks.

A diffuse loss of scalp hair often occurs without any obvious cause in women. Sometimes the magnitude of the complaint outweighs the actual observed loss. Presumably in these women either the observed increased rate of hair loss is matched by an increased rate of hair growth or the complaint is imaginary. In either case reassurance is required.

Where there is observable hair loss it should first be checked whether trauma could be the cause. Any persistent traction can cause hair loss. Severe systemic disease, some endocrine disorders (eg, hypothyroidism or a virilizing syndrome) and drugs can cause marked hair fall and reasonable care must be taken to exclude these possibilities.

It frequently happens that after investigation no cause is identified. In this case reassurance is justified, for in a large proportion of women with this problem their hair loss either remains static or recovers. In any event there are no effective treatments available at present for this condition, though some drugs that can stimulate hair growth are on trial.

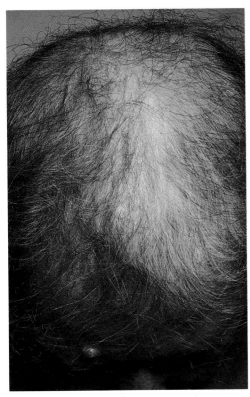

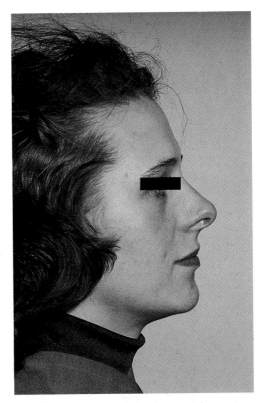

Androgenetic hair loss in women is quite common. It does not necessarily mean that there is a virilizing syndrome present. However, if there are other features of virilization, this possibility should be investigated. In women the condition is often more severe over the vertex than on either temple.

Mild temporal hair loss in a woman due to early androgenetic alopecia.

Alopecia areata

This is a common disorder in which hair growth suddenly ceases in circumscribed areas. This results in hair fall from these sites and the appearance of curious exclamation-mark-like hair stumps on the affected area. It most commonly occurs on the scalp but is also common in the beard area in men. Several such bald areas may appear together, or several patches may coalesce. Less commonly the whole scalp is affected, and rarely all the body hair may drop out at one go.

The outcome is almost totally unpredictable. Most small bald areas recover spontaneously after a few weeks or months – white hair regrowing first – but if the patient is atopic the outlook seems less good. When the hair loss has been extreme the outcome is even less certain – about one-third of cases seem to recover spontaneously after a few weeks, but in another one-third no regrowth ever seems to occur. Not a great deal is known about the cause but it seems to be autoimmune in origin and has associations with autoimmune thyroid disease. Many patients ask if it is caused by 'nerves' or stress. There is no evidence that it is but it seems that it may be precipitated by stress – most diseases can!

Treatment Application of potent topical corticosteroids to the affected sites seems to provoke regrowth in a small proportion but unfortunately the new hair tends to fall out again later in some cases. For widespread alopecia areata or alopecia totalis some

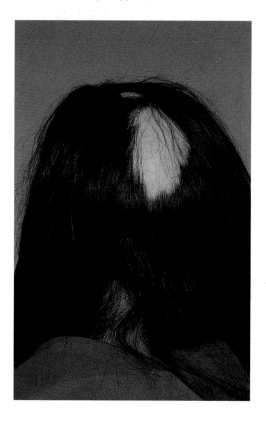

This woman has two patches of alopecia areata.

dermatologists have used short, sharp courses of systemic steroids lasting no more than a month. The results are only slightly better than from topical corticosteroids. In recent years various other treatments have been tried including sensitizing the skin with various chemical agents, such as diphencyprone. At the time of writing these seem only partially effective and some cause discomfort at the sites of treatment.

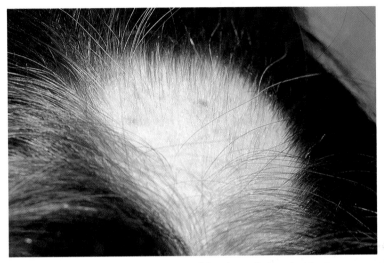

The prognosis for alopecia areata is good for the majority of patients. Regrowth is starting to occur in this bald patch.

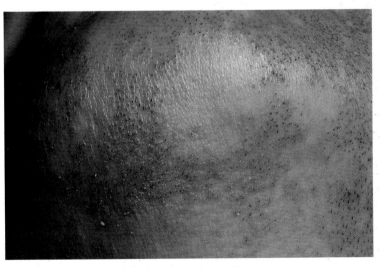

Typical alopecia areata of the beard area in a young man.

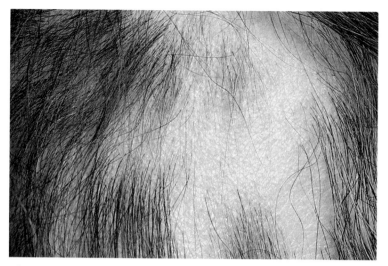

Alopecia areata affecting the scalp. A few wispy short hairs can be seen, representing regrowth.

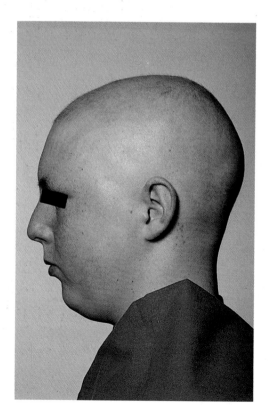

Alopecia totalis. The hair dropped out in this young man within a period of two or three weeks. Notice loss of hair from the eyebrows as well. The outlook in such patients is variable. If the hair does not regrow quickly then it is likely that the condition will persist.

Other causes

Permanent hair loss can result from any disorder that leads to destruction of the hair follicles. Some diseases seem to have a predilection for the scalp, such as lupus erythematosus and lichen planus. The inflammation that they cause results in damaged hair follicles and a patchy scarring alopecia. Trauma to the scalp will also cause a scarring type of alopecia.

HIRSUTISM

This is only a problem for women, because the media image of a woman is that she should be almost totally hair-free apart from her scalp. Nature recognizes no such media ideal and continues to allow normal women to develop some hair on the upper lip, chin, arms and legs. The areolae of the breasts and the lower abdomen may also be the sites of this inconvenient but normal hair growth.

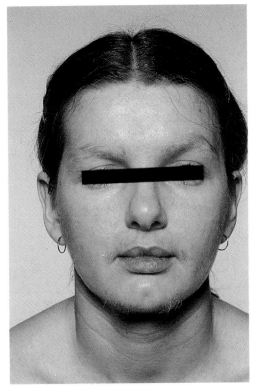

Hirsutism. This woman had excess hair growth on her upper lip, chin and pre-auricular region. Extensive investigation showed no endocrine abnormality.

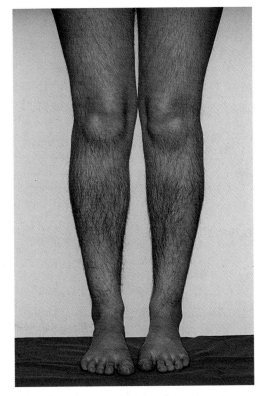

Legs of the same woman, showing male-pattern terminal hair growth on lower legs.

Diagnosis

When a woman presents complaining of excess hair, the practitioner has to consider various possibilities:

1. Is there actually excess hair present? Some who complain of excess hair have a disorder perception of their physical appearance and no real abnormality of hair growth.
2. If there does appear to be excess hair present, is this normal for the patient concerned or does it represent true hirsutism? There is a wide normal range, and some racial groups (Mediterranean types, for instance) and families have what is considered to be an unacceptable degree of hirsutism by conventional Western standards of the media ideal.
3. If the degree of hairiness present is frankly abnormal, is this due to virilization, drug treatment – such as with minoxidil (Loniten) – or common idiopathic hirsutism?

To sort out the cause it is usually necessary to take a full history, conduct a full physical examination and maybe determine the levels of testosterone and cortisone in the blood. For this reason, if there is any doubt as to the cause, the patient should be referred to a specialist.

Treatment

As far as local treatment is concerned this will depend on the severity and extent of the disorder.

Depilatories These are suitable for some patients, but not others. They can cause considerable soreness in some sensitive individuals – even if they are used according to instructions. Others object to using them on a regular basis.

Shaving Apart from on the legs, this is usually unacceptable.

Wax Many find depilating wax suitable for their needs.

Electrolysis This involves destruction of the hair follicles with an electric current. It is time-consuming (and costly if done privately) but its effect is permanent. It can leave slight puckering of the skin if not done well.

Hormones In some severely affected patients treatment with anti-androgens or other hormones is more appropriate. One anti-androgen known as cyproterone acetate has been combined with an oestrogen to make an oral preparation known as Dianette, which acts as a contraceptive pill. Although slightly helpful to some patients it does not seem to reverse the degree of hairiness in most women who use it for this purpose.

PRACTICAL POINTS

● Patients with male-pattern alopecia should be warned off quack cures.
● If reassurance is not sufficient, a toupee may be the answer for male patients who are worried about the effect of baldness on their appearance.
● Temporary hair loss may be caused by:
–Childbirth
–Alopecia areata
–Severe systemic disease
–Endocrine disorders
–Drugs.
● Hair loss in women may also be caused by:
–Androgenetic alopecia
–Trauma
–Scarring skin disease of the scalp.
● In many women who lose hair there is no obvious cause, and in this group the hair loss either stabilizes or recovers.
● Frankly abnormal hairiness in woman can be due to:
–Virilization
–Drugs, eg, minoxidil (Loniten)
–Idiopathic hirsutism.
● Treatments for excess body hair include:
–Depilatories
–Shaving
–Wax
–Electrolysis
–Hormone therapy.

25

Treatment of scabies and lice

BACKGROUND

Lice are more common than we like to think. They are no respecters of social status and unashamedly infest the middle classes. It is said that 10 per cent of the British population are infested with head lice at any one time. All lice are caught from direct contact – so combs and lavatory seats are the sources of infestation in polite conversation only! The best way to stop the beasts from spreading in the community is early diagnosis and treatment – and the removal of the social stigma of being infested.

LICE

Head lice

These are mainly a problem in children. When found, treatment should follow quickly. The older treatments with dichophane and gamma benzene hexachloride are no longer recommended as most lice are now resistant to these compounds. The pyrethroids – phenothrin (Full Marks shampoo) and Permethrin (Lyclear conditioner) are among the most popular and effective remedies for head lice. They should be used strictly according to the manufacturer's instructions. Another suitable treatment is with an organophosphorus compound such as malathion (Derbac, Prioderm). The head should be treated with malathion lotion and allowed to dry and shampooed and combed out twelve hours later. All members of the family and close contacts should be treated simultaneously. The shampoo may be an ordinary toilet shampoo, but preferably should be malathion based as well. An alternative treatment is with a carbamate-containing preparation (eg, Carylderm).

Pubic lice

Pretty much the same advice applies to pubic lice (crabs). An important aspect of the treatment of this condition is to make sure that all sexual contacts are treated simultaneously.

Body lice

These are the least common of the lice that live on humans. They differ from the other types in that they live in the clothing, particularly seams. They are mostly seen in the homeless and the very socially disadvantaged groups. Treatment must include fumigation of the clothing at a public fumigation centre.

SCABIES

Human scabies

There has been a major pandemic of scabies in recent years but it now grumbles on in the community at a somewhat more manageable level. Once again, awareness of the possibility of the condition and early treatment are all-important. As with pubic lice the disorder in adults is spread by sexual contact, so sexual partners (as well as family contacts) must be treated at the same time. Infants and children pick it up by crawling into bed with their parents or cuddling infested children or adults.

Benzyl benzoate application (eg, Ascabiol) and gamma benzene hexachloride (eg, Quellada) are appropriate treatment and failure is not usually due to resistance but inadequate compliance with instructions (or incorrect advice). An important aspect of treatment is that the whole body (apart from the head and neck) is treated with the application. An effective regimen includes a hot bath at the start and then two coatings of the application. Some specialists recommend a further application after 24 hours, and I agree with this approach. It is important that all household and sexual contacts are treated simultaneously. Patients should be warned that they may continue to itch for a few weeks after the infestation has been cured. Other effective treatments include malathion (Prioderm) and monosulfiram (Tetmosol).

Cat and dog scabies

This is not common and is not caused by the same mite as human scabies. The mite bites only at the site of contact and does not spread outside. Treatment should be directed at the pet and a trip to the veterinarian is to be recommended.

PRACTICAL POINTS

- **Head lice and pubic lice**
  These should be treated promptly with a modern compound such as malathion (Derbac, Prioderm or Permethrin or phenothrin scalp treatment).
- **Body lice**
  Treatment must include fumigation of clothing.
- **Scabies**
  This should be treated with benzyl benzoate application or gamma benzene hexachloride (Ascabiol or Quellada), applied to the whole body, apart from the head and neck, on at least two occasions.
- Those who have been in close contact with sufferers from all these infestations must also be treated.

26

When to refer for specialist opinion

BACKGROUND

A practitioner's referring threshold is specific to him or herself and to the medical environment in which he or she practises. It also differs with the category of disease in question and according to the specialist facilities available. It is not the aim of this chapter to recommend uniformity or to lay down any set of rules. Its intent is to point out those situations in which for one reason or another a specialist opinion may be helpful and useful with regard to diagnosis, treatment, reassurance or future management of a patient.

RINGWORM

The problem of incorrect diagnosis and treatment

A frequent cause for confusion among practitioners is ringworm. I cannot count the number of patients with simple intertrigo of the groins who have been treated mistakenly with a succession of topical antifungal agents by colleagues in various types of practice. Similarly patients with ringworm who have been treated inappropriately with a succession of topical corticosteroids still present at skin clinics. When treated with corticosteroids in this way the ringworm takes on an unusual appearance. It becomes less red and scaly, its borders become less distinct but the whole of the patch tends to enlarge. This atypical appearance has become sufficiently frequently seen to be known as 'tinea incognito' because it is in disguise!

It is easy to criticize these incorrect treatments but not so easy to give simple pointers as to how to avoid making them. In fact although dermatologists may make the clinical diagnosis of ringworm or dermatitis with greater ease and confidence than other physicians, they will usually take specimens of skin scales for culture to make absolutely sure. There are some easily detectable signs, though, which help to distinguish the clinical features of ringworm from other common scaling dermatoses. They include:

1. The presence of a well-defined rounded edge and asymmetrical distribution of the rash in ringworm.
2. The edge may also be redder and slightly more raised than the centre of the lesion.

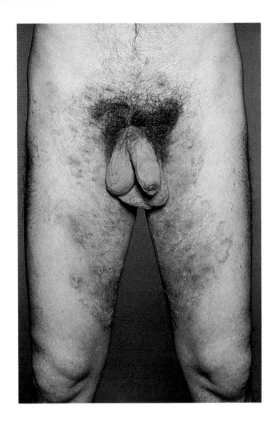

Very extensive and inflamed ringworm affecting both thighs and groins due to misdiagnosis and application of betamethasone-17-valerate (Betnovate) ointment over a period of two months. The original problem was a small scaling patch on the left thigh which the practitioner thought was psoriasis.

3. A history of previous similar episodes of the rash as well as rash elsewhere will tend to support a diagnosis of dermatitis.

None of these features are invariable.

It really is very easy to make a mistake. I remember only too well a pleasant elderly lady with systemic sclerosis who developed an odd scaly erythema on her forehead and trunk. It was thought that her rash was basically dermatitis and coincidental to her connective tissue disease; she was treated with topical corticosteroids. Her rash spread and worsened and it was only after a few weeks of the wrong treatment that the penny dropped and she was correctly diagnosed as having ringworm.

When to refer

If there are facilities available locally it is easy to scrape a few scales gently off the lesion with a blunt scalpel, put them between two glass slides or in a small envelope and send them to the local pathology laboratory. If this is not possible and there is any doubt about the diagnosis it is much better to refer the patient to the skin clinic than to treat blindly.

While the patient is waiting for an appointment the safest topical agent to use is a simple emollient cream. Opinions differ as to the usefulness of antifungal/corticosteroid

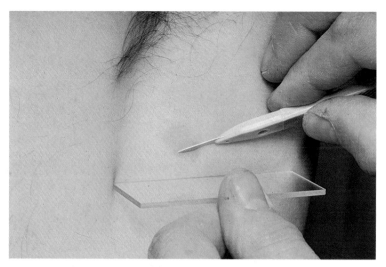

The reddened scaly area in this young man's armpits is being gently scraped with a scalpel blade. The skin scrapings are allowed to fall onto a glass slide held beneath. When sufficient scales have been collected, another slide is placed on top and taped in position to hold the scales on the slide. The preparation can then be sent to the laboratory for examination for fungal mycelium.

combinations. They should *not* be used instead of making a diagnosis. To do so is to court disaster and in my view is the antithesis of good medical practice. Combinations certainly have a place, but only after a diagnosis has been made (see page 171).

DERMATITIS AND PSORIASIS

When to refer for diagnosis?

Dermatitis and psoriasis are both red and scaly and can affect similar anatomical sites. A common clinical situation in which they may be difficult to distinguish is involvement of the palms and/or soles with a persistent scaling eruption. As skin disease of these areas causes considerable embarrassment, discomfort and disablement it is important to make the correct diagnosis as quickly as possible and commence the right treatment. This may involve patch tests to potential contact sensitizers and skin biopsy – both of which should be performed by specialists (see Chapter 38).

Early referral to a dermatologist can be very helpful for this type of patient. This should not be taken to mean that every patient with scaly palms and soles who is seen in the skin clinic will be rapidly diagnosed and healed. Every dermatologist has a group of chronic patients who attend on many occasions and for whom the diagnosis and treatment change with each visit. This type of skin disorder can be intrinsically difficult for even the most skilled specialist. It is nonetheless important to obtain the best opinion and advice on management at an early stage in the disease. If very little can be done to give substantial help then at least the patient and practitioner know the score.

Atopic dermatitis: when to refer for treatment?

This can be the most frustrating and difficult disorder to treat (see also Chapter 15). The more severely affected patients are obviously in great physical discomfort, with their lives in tatters. The parents are anxious and distressed and often the whole family is tense and disturbed. When the usual remedies such as emollients and mild cortico-steroids are not giving relief it is time to obtain skilled advice. Progression to a more potent corticosteroid for use in the long term is not the answer and can be hazardous (see page 170). If this type of preparation is needed for these patients it is as well to have the assistance of a dermatologist who will know its advantages and disadvantages.

Patients with severe atopic dermatitis are often best helped by a period of treatment as in-patients. They may respond rapidly to a few days of hospitalization, with only minor modifications to their treatment regimen. Whether this is due to removal from an environment containing antigens to which they are sensitized and/or stress, or is due to the rest and care available in hospital, is not known.

Atopic dermatitis is a very common disease and luckily most patients are only mildly affected. If the practitioner is confident as to the diagnosis and has the interest and ability to ring the changes in treatment when required, and no special problems arise, then there is no point to referral. Sometimes parents want a second opinion or a chat with a special-ist about management and then consultation with a dermatologist should be arranged.

Psoriasis: when to refer for treatment?

When psoriasis is extensive (say more than 15 per cent of the body surface) or is on particularly awkward areas (face, palms, soles or genitalia) a dermatologist's advice should be sought. Some of the treatments now available for severe psoriasis really require hospital clinic supervision (see also Chapter 19). Treatment with methotrexate, etretinate/acitretin (Tigason, Neotigason) or cyclosporin or by any form of ultraviolet light (especially PUVA – photochemotherapy with A-type ultraviolet light) has to be carefully regulated. Even when psoriasis is less extensive, advice concerning the best form of topical treatment may be helpful. This is especially the case if the moderately potent or potent corticosteroids are contemplated. Psoriasis is a persistent or relapsing disorder and these applications can be damaging (see page 170) especially in the long term if not used with care.

When an apparently typical lesion of psoriasis remains stubbornly unchanged or slowly enlarges on the legs or trunk of an elderly person the diagnosis should be questioned. Bowen's disease (a form of carcinoma-in-situ – intraepidermal epithelioma – see page 188) may present in this way and needs early attention.

OTHER SCALING RASHES

It goes without saying that whenever there is real difficulty with diagnosis then the opinion of a dermatologist should be obtained. As many ex-medical students will remember, there are large numbers of rare, red and scaling rashes which cause hours of hot debate and can puzzle even dermatologists. Occasionally a lymphoma of the skin – mycosis fungoides – will present as a persistent psoriasis-like rash of the trunk.

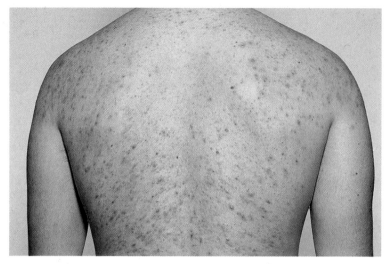

Extensive and severe acne affecting almost the whole back like this is probably best referred for dermatological opinion.

Treatment for this disorder has improved but has become very specialized, so that the earlier these patients are seen now the better their outlook may be. Some scaling rashes are signs of serious internal disease (see Chapter 37) and here too, early diagnosis can be very important.

ACNE

Obviously dermatologists cannot see every patient with acne. Most people experience some acne at some stage but only a relatively small proportion of the population have it badly enough to require any formal treatment. The time to refer patients with acne for specialist opinion is when, despite the best efforts of the practitioner, the disease is worsening and the sufferer is becoming anxious and depressed because of it. Do not expect topical treatments or systemic tetracycline to work overnight – it may be two months or even longer before any improvement occurs in the condition.

When the face and back/and or chest are involved at the same time, and the lesions are large and painful, then it is probably best to refer the patient for dermatological opinion at an early stage as some form of specialized treatment may be necessary.

BLISTERING DISORDERS

When a generalized blistering disease develops (see Chapter 35) then the attention of a specialist is urgently required.

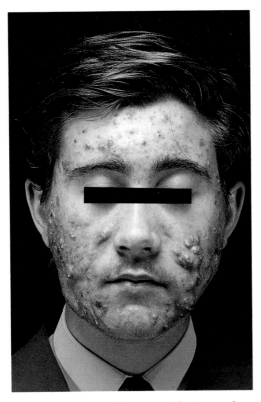

Very severe acne, with large cystic lesions on the jaw line and cheeks. Luckily this young man's condition responded to specialist treatment and he ended with very little scarring.

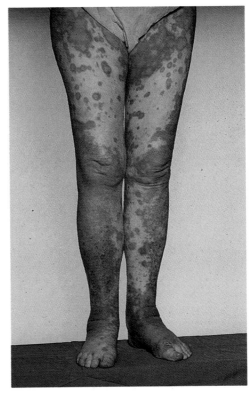

Extensive erythema multiforme. This rash occurred after herpes simplex infection. Many of the lesions develop blisters and become eroded.

Pemphigoid and erythema multiforme

These disorders may appear quite abruptly and patients need specialized nursing and treatment from a dermatologist as soon as possible.

Dermatitis herpetiformis

This is an itchy, vesicular and blistering disease which is not usually dramatic in its onset but gives rise to distressing itchiness. It responds well to dapsone (Maloprim) but will need to be treated by a gluten-free diet in the long term as this may reduce or eliminate the need for the drug.

Pemphigus

This potentially fatal disease may start insidiously but can also present acutely. It may start with erosive areas in the mouth. Distinguishing between these and other blistering disorders is a skilled affair and requires histological examination of the skin and immunofluorescence tests.

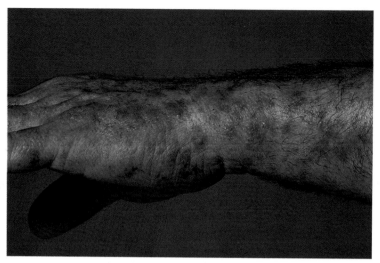

Another example of severe erythema multiforme.

The blistering disorders

Disease	Site of blister in skin	Major clinical features
● Pemphigus	Intraepidermal	Thin-walled blisters or erosions affecting any area of skin and mucosae. Prior to steroids was frequently fatal.
● Pemphigoid	Subepidermal	Sudden onset of blistering on any area of skin. Blisters often large and blood filled. Mostly affects elderly patients. Remits after variable period.
● Dermatitis herpetiformis	Subepidermal	Itchy blisters and vesicles. Knees, elbows, scalp and buttocks mainly affected. Tends to persist.
● Erythema multiforme	Subepidermal	Sudden onset of reddened areas on which blisters occur. Mucosae often involved. Can be provoked by drugs and some infections. Multiple attacks may occur.
● Epidermolysis bullosa	Mostly subepidermal but some forms are intraepidermal	A group of rare inherited disorders. Simple forms are nonscarring but dystrophic forms cause dreadful scarring.
● Porphyria cutanea tarda	Subepidermal	Metabolic disorder, probably inherited. Blisters occur on light-exposed skin.
● Herpes simplex and herpes zoster	Intraepidermal	Viral diseases which small vesicles grouped in characteristic ways.

WARTY LESIONS

Viral warts

Ordinary viral warts are extremely common (see Chapter 22). Most people have had, have or will have these small viral tumours. Fortunately the great majority disappear spontaneously within weeks or months. Patience and reassurance should be the ingredients of treatment. If these do not suffice, a keratolytic agent containing salicylic acid or a destructive substance such as formaldehyde or podophyllin extract can be used. Referral of patients with these lesions is only recommended if:

1. There are several lesions that are persistent and have resisted simple treatments.
2. There are a vast number of lesions and it seems possible that there is a serious underlying immunological defect.
3. There are some warts that are large, persistent and embarrassing, and electrocautery or cryotherapy seem to be indicated.
4. There is some doubt as to the diagnosis.

Seborrhoeic warts

Ordinary viral warts have to be distinguished from simple seborrhoeic warts which usually start to make their appearance in the fifth and sixth decades (see Chapter 36). Seborrhoeic warts are usually pigmented, the shade varying from light fawn to dark brown and black. These mostly do not need attention unless they are very large or become inflamed. Sometimes they occur in large numbers and are an embarrassment, and referral for advice as to treatment may be required.

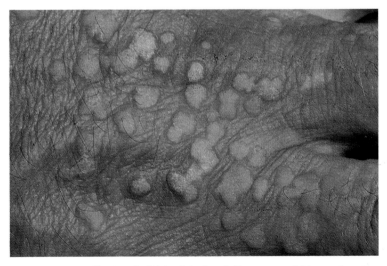

Extensive warts affecting the back of the hand. Treatment of this number of warts is always a problem.

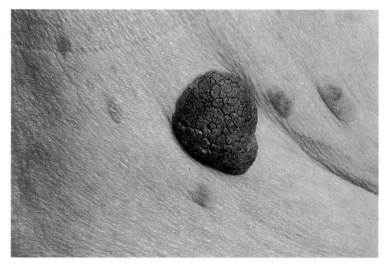

Multiple seborrhoeic warts. Some of these lesions get in the way and catch in clothing.

Solar keratoses and small skin cancers

As their name suggests, solar keratoses occur on the light-exposed sites (see Chapter 11). They are preneoplastic in the broadest sense of the term but only progress to squamous cell carcinoma extremely rarely (perhaps in 0.01 per cent of cases). Their main importance is that they signify solar damage of the kind that can result in a malignant lesion. Solar keratoses are usually found in the elderly although they may occur at an earlier age if there has been a great deal of sun exposure in the past. They are much commoner in the fair-skinned, who have little protective pigmentation.

Small skin cancers (squamous cell epithelioma and Bowen's disease) may also be difficult to distinguish from other warty lesions. If there is any question, refer.

Genital warts

Warty lesions on the genitalia probably always require the opinion of a specialist. The majority are simple viral warts, but tragedies occur if syphilitic warts or squamous cell carcinoma are not diagnosed at an early stage.

PIGMENTED LESIONS

Whatever else the practitioner may forget of his undergraduate training in dermatology, the danger of malignant melanoma usually remains well in mind (see Chapter 36). Delay in the referral of a suspected malignant melanoma is usually either due to the patient presenting late because of fear or ignorance, or an office bungle. In few other skin disorders is early referral so vital to the well-being of the patient. If a pigmented lesion

enlarges, changes in colour, ulcerates or bleeds the patient should be seen by a dermatologist at the first opportunity. Dermatologists would prefer to see a hundred patients
referred to their clinics who did not have the disease than one patient with the disease
in an advanced stage who has been referred late and for whom there is a bad prognosis. The danger signals of a melanoma are:

1. History of change in colour, increase in size and surface changes including
   scaling, crusting and bleeding.
2. Irregularity in colour (variegation).
3. Irregularity of margin.
4. A lesion more than 1 cm in diameter.

PRACTICAL POINTS

● **Ringworm**
1. Refer to specialist diagnosis if there are no local pathology laboratory facilities and when there is doubt as to diagnosis.
2. Do not use potent topical corticosteroid preparations until a diagnosis has been made.

● **Dermatitis**
Refer:
1. Patients presenting with persistent scaling eruption of palms and/or soles.
2. Severe atopics if prescribed treatments appear not to be working.

● **Psoriasis**
Refer:
1. As Dermatitis 1. above
2. When psoriasis affects over 15 per cent of body.
3. When on awkward areas and causes disability.
4. When there is any doubt as to diagnosis.
5. When condition does not respond to simple treatments.

● **Acne**
Refer:
1. If patient is depressed by unsuccessful treatment.
2. When large, painful lesions appear concurrently on face and back and/or chest.

● **Blistering disorders**
Always refer patients with widespread blistering disorders such as:
–Pemphigoid and erythema multiforme
–Dermatitis herpetiformis
–Pemphigus.

● **Warts**
Refer:
1. If persistent, large or inflamed.
2. If they appear in vast numbers.
3. If there is any doubt over diagnosis.
4. If they are genital.

● **Pigmented lesions**
Always refer if they:
1. Enlarge.
2. Change colour.
3. Ulcerate.
4. Bleed.

27

Advice on the use of topical corticosteroids

BACKGROUND

It is frequently stated by dermatologists that the introduction of topical corticosteroids in the 1950s heralded a new era in dermatology. I believe this is an uncritical view and that although these drugs have helped many patients, they have much to answer for. Essentially, corticosteroids are suppressive to all types of inflammation and are a sophisticated type of symptomatic treatment. Surprisingly, during the thirty-odd years in which they have been in general use we have not gained a full understanding of the way in which this suppression works and there is as yet no rational basis for using a particular corticosteroid to treat a particular type of inflammation.

Whenever they are used to treat symptoms and signs of skin disease the prescriber must not 'suppress' further thoughts about treating the disorder and should appreciate that their function is to buy time. It cannot be emphasized too strongly that they are in no sense curative. In many instances when application ceases the underlying disorder returns, sometimes with increased vigour – the so-called rebound effect. Of course this may not be the case when the skin disease for which the corticosteroid is being applied is self-limiting, such as allergic contact dermatitis (see Chapter 34) or sunburn (see Chapter 11).

THERAPEUTIC EFFECTS

The vehicle in which the corticosteroid is formulated often has a therapeutic effect itself. Bland creams and ointments (especially those containing white soft paraffin) have a fascinating array of pharmacological effects and may provide considerable relief without the addition of a corticosteroid. This is especially true in the chronic dermatoses and it is always worth prescribing a bland emollient in the first place. If it does little good at least it will do no harm.

When a patient's skin disorder improves after application of a topical corticosteroid there are four possible explanations:

1. The disease was getting better anyway, and the application had no real biological effect.
2. The preparation was effective by virtue of its bland emollient properties and not its corticosteroid properties.
3. The fact of treatment itself and the care exhibited by the physician exerted a true placebo effect.
4. The beneficial effect was caused by the anti-inflammatory properties of the corticosteroid content.

Clearly one has to be careful before accepting the relief of symptoms as due to the corticosteroid content of the preparation.

Topical corticosteroids need not be applied more than twice per day, and in most cases need only be given once daily. More frequent application gives no added beneficial effect. The patient should be advised to apply only the thinnest smear; to apply more gives no additional benefit and is merely wasteful.

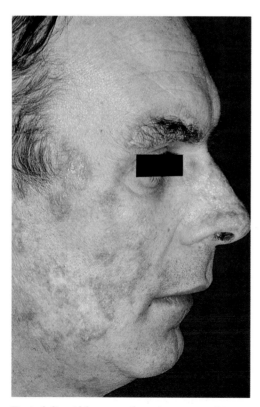

Typical discoid lupus erythematosus – a resistant dermatosis that should respond to a high-potency corticosteroid application. Note the pale scarring at the centre of some of the lesions. If these lesions occur in the hairy areas, the destruction causes hair loss, as in this man's eyebrow. Individual inflamed areas are raised, red and scaly.

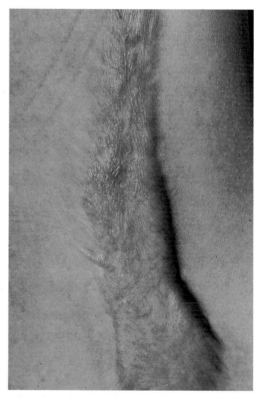

Keloid scar of the upper arm in a young woman who had injured herself at the site some three months previously. This would respond either to application of a high-potency corticosteroid or intralesional injection of a suitable corticosteroid preparation.

POTENCY

It has become fashionable to group corticosteroids according to their potency. A table of the different groups with examples is given below.

The most potent should only be used by those who are experienced both with the natural history of the skin disease they are treating and with the full range of actions and side-effects of the particular preparation. They should only be employed for the uncommon and very resistant dermatoses – such as severe discoid lupus erythematosus, alopecia areata and keloid scars.

The least potent are quite useful for the dermatitic group of disorders. Hydrocortisone preparations of one sort or another are often all that are required for patients with atopic dermatitis (see Chapter 15) or patients with dermatitis affecting the hands (see Chapter 16).

In general, the most appropriate corticosteroid is the weakest necessary to control the disorder treated. It is perfectly reasonable to give a moderately potent or potent corticosteroid preparation for the worst areas and a weak preparation to the other less badly affected zones. If this is done, it is important to make it crystal clear to the patient which goes where.

Particular care is needed when corticosteroids are prescribed for the face and flexural areas, as these sites are susceptible to skin-thinning and masked infection (see opposite). For these reasons potent and very potent corticosteroids should not be used on these areas. Potent steroids are also more likely to cause stretch marks in pregnant women and adolescents, especially over the upper limbs and on the lower abdomen. Their use should be restricted in these groups.

Potency of some common corticosteroids

Weak	Hydrocortisone preparations (Dioderm, Dio-Cort)
	Clobetasone butyrate (Eumovate)
Moderately potent	Fluocortolone (Ultradil, Ultralanum)
	Flurandrenolone (Haelan)
Potent	Betamethasone valerate (Betnovate)
	Fluocinolone acetonide (Synalar)
Very potent	Clobetasol propionate (Dermovate)

HARMFUL SIDE-EFFECTS OF CORTICOSTEROIDS

Prescribing a corticosteroid application for an inflammatory skin disorder is no substitute for making a diagnosis. Many types of inflammation are improved by their use, but for some skin disorders the use of corticosteroids is quite incorrect.

Aggravating infection

Infections are a case in point. Treatment of a ringworm infection with corticosteroids leads to considerable problems. The inflammation is reduced but the infection remains, and in fact spreads. This may produce a bizarre appearance and ringworm of quite dramatic extent, which has come to be known as tinea incognito, as its characteristic features have become disguised (see page 154). The sharp outline and scaling surface of typical ringworm gives way to a diffuse pink area which is not very itchy. This area tends to become lumpy and more inflamed when the corticosteroids are stopped, so in many cases they continue to be used, even though it is obvious that the area being treated is gradually spreading. Clearly the way to avoid falling into this trap is to prescribe corticosteroids only when one is confident of the diagnosis.

Skin-thinning

Corticosteroids, particularly the most potent ones, cause skin-thinning. The skin-thinning may be very marked, as for example in a patient of mine who had used a fluocinolone acetonide preparation for 6 years on her left leg for an ill-defined dermatitic condition. When corticosteroids are used for long periods of time the veins can easily be seen

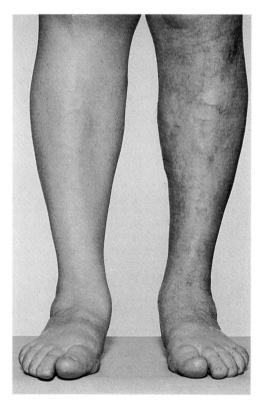

This patient's left lower leg looks thinner than the right. Superficial veins are more easily seen and the skin is pinker. Palpation confirmed that there was severe thinning of the skin. This was due to fluocinolone acetonide cream (Synalar) used twice daily on the leg for a period of six years.

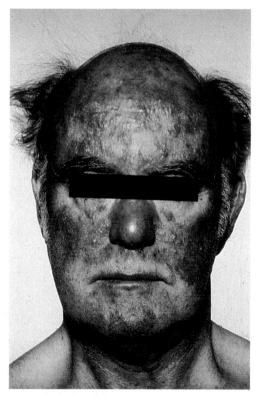

Marked redness of the face together with typical rosacea papules. This man's rosacea was considerably aggravated by the use of a preparation containing betamethasone-17-valerate (Betnovate).

through the skin, which becomes paper-thin. Crimson stains (ecchymoses) may appear, similar to those that occur in the sun-exposed skin of the elderly. The thinned skin becomes prone to injury and heals poorly.

The colour of the affected skin is variable, but where there is a good blood supply may be quite pink. This effect is due to the increased visibility of the underlying microvasculature which is nearer the surface than usual. One the face this pinkness may be the main feature and becomes a startling, clown-like red over the cheeks. Happily, skin-thinning and colour changes are slowly reversible, recovering if application of corticosteroids is stopped.

Stretch marks

In some sites – notably the thighs, upper arms and abdomen – unsightly broad stretch marks (striae) may occur. Unfortunately the stretch marks are not reversible. Particular care should be taken in giving potent corticosteroid preparations to young women, as they are especially prone to develop these breaks in the integrity of the dermal connective tissue and also find them quite disturbing.

Adrenal failure due to absorption

Another danger is from absorption of the corticosteroids through the skin and into the blood. Use of more than 75 g per week of a potent corticosteroid preparation for more than two or three weeks produces some degree of pituitary–adrenal axis suppression

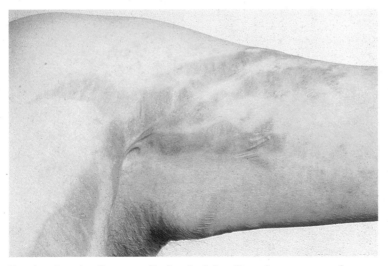

Broad, ugly striae distensae affecting the left axilla and upper arm and adjoining chest wall in a man treated with various potent corticosteroid preparations for psoriasis over a period of a year. These striae will never entirely fade. Considerable care should be taken in treating the flexural areas with potent steroids.

Dangers of topical corticosteroids

- Absorption of corticosteroid into circulation sufficient to cause pituitary–adrenal axis suppression and, rarely, even adrenal failure.
- Absorption of corticosteroid into circulation sufficient to cause a Cushingoid state. This is rare.
- Skin-thinning from local absorption. On the face this can lead to bizarrely reddened facial features. In the flexures it can cause unpleasant purple striae.
- Suppression of local inflammatory response to infection of the skin. Can lead to the infection spreading and give rise to difficulties in diagnosis due to strange appearances, eg, tinea incognito.
- Rebound of treated disorder after stopping treatment to worse state than that originally treated. This is particularly a problem with psoriasis – may even precipitate the pustular form of the disease.
- Occasionally acne-type spots, increase in hairiness and slight decrease in skin pigmentation may occur.

which causes a detectable reduction in the plasma cortisol levels. If this suppression persists then adrenal atrophy may occur, with the possibility of adrenal failure if the topical steroid is suddenly stopped or some type of severe stress occurs. This is very uncommon but as some tragedies have been recorded after liberal use of the more potent corticosteroids all prescribers of these drugs must be aware of the potential hazard.

To complicate matters there are a number of variables which make it difficult to predict accurately just when danger is present:

1. The potency of the corticosteroid used.
2. The area over which it is used.
3. The length of time over which it is given.
4. The barrier presented by the skin to the absorption of the drug.

It is difficult to predict the degree of penetration through abnormal skin, save to say that it is increased. Bandaging the skin with airtight materials increases penetration. Plastic film occlusion was used at one time to increase the suppressive effect of corticosteroids; it is not now recommended. A reasonable rule is to be aware of the danger in a patient with skin lesions occupying more than 20 per cent of the body area, who is being treated with an undiluted potent or moderately potent steroid for four weeks or more.

In psoriasis

Corticosteroids should not be used for the majority of patients with plaque-type psoriasis because of the danger of absorption (see Chapter 19). In addition, many dermatologists believe that it is possible to precipitate pustular psoriasis by using topical corticosteroids on ordinary plaque-type psoriasis. However, psoriasis of the flexures, scalp (and face) and very occasionally elsewhere may at times need to be treated with weak or moderately potent corticosteroids.

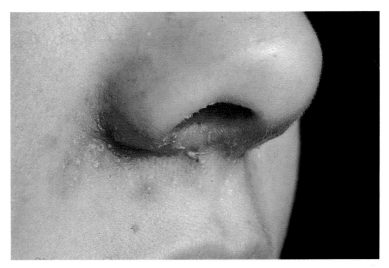

Typical seborrhoeic dermatitis affecting the nasolabial groove. A corticosteroid preparation combined with an antibacterial agent may be more effective in this type of disorder than a plain corticosteroid.

In rosacea and perioral dermatitis

The possible danger of the use of corticosteroids on the face has already been mentioned. It is briefly mentioned again here to emphasize the hazards of treating patients with rosacea or perioral dermatitis with topical corticosteroids. Both these conditions are made worse with these topical agents.

CORTICOSTEROID/ANTIMICROBIAL COMBINATIONS

There is a large number of proprietary preparations in which corticosteroids are combined with either an antibiotic or a nonantibiotic antimicrobial substance. They are sometimes promoted on the basis of their availability to cope with secondary infection, although this is not a problem for many patients with skin disease. They do appear useful for some individuals with seborrhoeic dermatitis and others with infected atopic dermatitis (see Chapter 15). It should be remembered that certain antibiotics may cause allergic contact dermatitis after topical application (see Chapter 34).

PRACTICAL POINTS

- Corticosteroids suppress symptoms but do not cure skin disease.
- The skin lesions may flare to become worse than before treatment when corticosteroids are stopped.
- The weakest beneficial strength should be prescribed.
- A thin smear twice a day is sufficient dosage.
- Corticosteroids should not be prescribed before making a diagnosis or for:
  –Infections (including ringworm)
  –Most types of psoriasis
  –Rosacea
  –Perioral dermatitis.
- The possibility of adrenal failure following adrenal suppression caused by corticosteroid absorption should be borne in mind. This applies when treating a patient with extensive lesions with moderate or potent corticosteroids for over four weeks. Rarely, a Cushingoid state can result.

28

Advice on the use of antimicrobials and antibiotics

BACKGROUND

In popular imagination, skin disorders are dirty and are due to contact with something or someone dirty. This folk myth probably has its roots in a time when most skin disease was due to infection and infestation, and when contact with someone with a rash was hazardous. It goes without saying that these beliefs about skin diseases are now totally inappropriate. Regrettably these feelings (and the accompanying prejudices) live on – even in the minds of some doctors. An oozing eruption which finally crusts is more often due to dermatitis inflammation rather than skin infection. The appearance of pus spots does not necessarily mean infection – pustular psoriasis and acne pustules are not the result of microbial invasion.

TOPICAL USE OF ANTIMICROBIALS AND ANTIBIOTICS

Unwanted effects

In general, antibiotics and other antimicrobial drugs are used more frequently than necessary. The problem often starts before the patient reaches the door. Dettol, TCP and Cetavlex may have been obtained at the local store and liberally applied to an inflamed area regardless as to whether acne, dermatitis, psoriasis or syphilis is the cause. Not only do these medicaments do little good, they often do considerable harm by irritating an already sore area or causing added allergic contact hypersensitivity.

Prescribed antibiotics too can cause these unwanted effects and lead to worse problems than the one for which they were originally prescribed. Penicillin is particularly liable to do this (thankfully it is hardly ever used topically), but neomycin and chloramphenicol (which are) may also cause a reaction.

Another major disadvantage is the bacterial resistance that the use of topical antibiotics engenders. This is a hazard not only in the patient's own environment but also in the community at large. If there is not some control over the use of these drugs on the skin there is a real danger of the spread of multiresistant micro-organisms causing disease that will not respond to most of the conventionally used antibiotics.

Ideally, antimicrobial drugs should only be used when it has been shown that a micro-organism is responsible for or is contributing to the disorder – and then only when it is

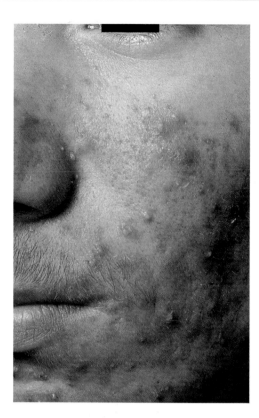

Acne. Note there are several pustules on the skin. These pustular lesions do not contain pathogenic bacteria.

known that the particular micro-organism is sensitive to the antimicrobial in question. (There is no place, however, for topical antimicrobial measures in such deep-rooted infections as cellulitis or carbuncles or severe acute infections such as erysipelas.)

Conditions suitable for treatment

Acne There are some circumstances when the rules may be slightly bent. Acne is one such case. In this disease it is believed that there is some clinical benefit to be derived from reducing the numbers of bacteria on the skin, because this leads to a decrease in the fat-splitting activity of the resident bacteria in the hair follicles. Antibacterial facial washes containing hexachlorophane and topical agents containing antibiotics, benzoyl peroxide and hydroxyquinolone are thought to act in this way. All antibacterial preparations seem to offer some benefit to patients with inflamed acne.

Ringworm Rashes in the flexures, particularly the groin, are often misdiagnosed as being due to ringworm, and antifungal agents prescribed inappropriately. Beware of the attitude that admits that the clinical diagnosis might be wrong and that it is better to prescribe something that will cover all eventualities. There is no substitute for making the right diagnosis. If the diagnosis is impossible to reach for one reason or another it is

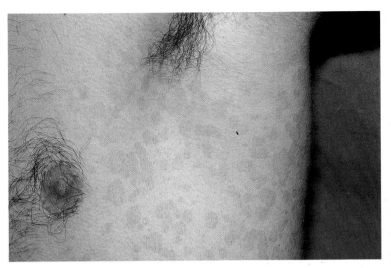

Pityriasis versicolor (tinea versicolor). Notice the spotty depigmentation of this man's skin. Even in Caucasian individuals the depigmentation from this mild fungal disorder is easily seen and may sometimes be a problem.

correct to give symptomatic treatment but incorrect to give potent suppressive therapies that may confuse the picture and lead to subsequent difficulties.

When a positive diagnosis of ringworm has been made there is little to beat the modern imidazole group of antimicrobial agents for effective and trouble-free therapy. These include miconazole (Daktarin, Monistat), clotrimazole (Canesten) and econazole (Ecostatin). In addition, terbinafine (Lamisil) and amorolfine (Loceryl) have been shown to be effective topical agents. Systemic therapies for stubborn and extensive ringworm infections include griseofulvin, itraconazole, ketoconazole and terbinafine.

Pityriasis versicolor This mild condition of the trunk, which is due to overgrowth of a normal yeast-like denizen of the hair follicles (known as malassezia furfur), also responds to the imidazole group of drugs. It responds too to selenium disulphide shampoo (Selsun) and to 20 per cent sodium thiosulphate solution. Systemic itraconazole has also proved safe and effective.

Secondary infections The question of secondary infection frequently arises in herpes zoster (shingles) and atopic dermatitis (see Chapter 15) as well as in gravitational ulcers (see Chapter 23) and numerous other disorders. In my view the traditional advice that antibiotic prophylaxis is bad medicine still holds true. If antibacterial measures are required for this purpose, it is probably better to use nonantibiotic antimicrobial compounds, though the philosophy remains the same. To be fair, the situation in seborrhoeic dermatitis and some patients with atopic dermatitis may differ slightly because there is genuine argument as to whether bacteria play some role in the development and perpetuation of these disorders.

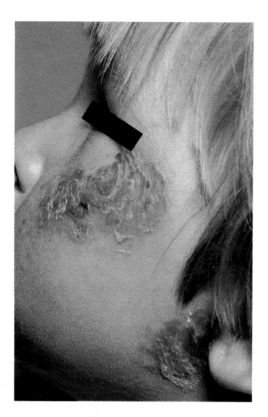

Impetigo of the facial skin in a young boy. The lesions blistered, became exudative and then developed a golden crust. Such patients respond well to systemic antibiotics of the penicillin type.

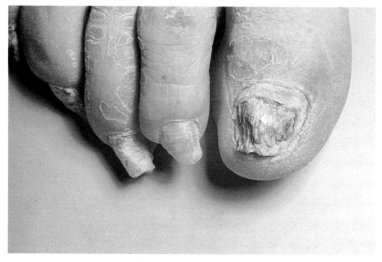

Chronic ringworm affecting the toe-nails. Affected nails are yellow, thickened and crumbling. Systemic treatment with griseofulvin, terbinafine or ketoconazole is necessary.

SYSTEMIC ANTIMICROBIALS

In many cases when an antimicrobial drug is indicated for a skin disorder it is more appropriate to use a systemic agent rather than a topical one.

In impetigo, which is caused by staphylococci and streptococci, the disorder responds best to systemic penicillin (or another antibiotic). Local treatment may be confined to washing off the crusts and short-term use of an antimicrobial – such as miconazole (Daktarin or Monistat) – to inhibit the local spread of the disorder before the penicillin has had a chance to act.

Ringworm of the nails can be annoyingly resistant to treatment. It just does not respond to topical agents and requires protracted treatment with griseofulvin (Fulcin, Grisovin), ketoconazole (Nizoral) or terbinafine (Lamisil) by mouth. Treatment with these agents does not unfortunately guarantee success.

Finally, rosacea and perioral dermatitis are two facial skin diseases that generally respond well to oral tetracycline (see Chapter 33).

PRACTICAL POINTS

- Not all pustular eruptions are signs of infections that require antimicrobial treatment.
- Topical antibiotics – especially penicillin, neomycin and chloramphenicol – may cause skin sensitization and allergic contact dermatitis.
- Indiscriminate use of antimicrobials may lead to the spread of multiresistant bacteria.
- Antibiotic prophylaxis against secondary infection is not recommended.

29

Tar, dithranol and other traditional remedies

TAR

Tar is the thick oily material left after the distillation of coal or wood. It contains literally thousands of different organic compounds, including the paraffin waxes and various phenolic substances. The composition varies according to the type of distillation and the material distilled, but there is also some variability from batch to batch even when these two factors are constant. Most preparations for use on the skin contain concentrations of 1–6 per cent, but a crude coal tar preparation is also available. Unfortunately the strength of this varies somewhat with the supplier.

Conditions suited to treatment

Tar ointments or tar pastes are of most use in psoriasis and chronic dermatitic rashes, though why tar should be effective in these conditions is as mysterious as how it came to be used in the first place. These preparations are particularly helpful for areas of thickened and itchy dermatitis and thick patches of stubborn psoriasis. Sometimes tar is used together with ultraviolet light, which seems to enhance its action. Creams and gels containing tar are sometimes helpful for patients with atopic dermatitis or other forms of more widespread dermatitic rash; liquid formulations of tar (eg, Polytar liquid) are particularly helpful for patients with psoriasis, both as additives to the bath and as shampoos.

Unwanted side-effects

Tar preparations don't suit everybody, and can cause irritation of the skin. They can also cause a type of acne-like inflammation of the hair follicles (folliculitis). Unfortunately most of the available tar preparations are messy and make unpleasant marks on bedclothes, towels and clothes. They also have a strong characteristic smell. To avoid these disadvantages the treated site can be bandaged with cotton gauze. Some proprietary tar preparations, such as tar cream (Clinitar), are less troublesome but haven't entirely done away with the staining or smell. In its crude form, tar is undoubtedly carcinogenic in small mammals. It contains benzpyrene and dimethylbenzanthracene. However, despite intense searching no excess cancer has been found in patients treated with tars for skin disorders. Clearly, there is a potential risk but it must be very small.

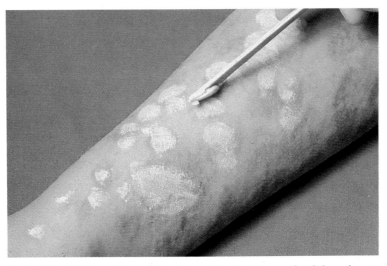

Application of dithranol to patches of psoriasis. In this case the dithranol preparation used is dithranol in Lassar's paste. Notice that the material is only applied to the sites of the lesions.

DITHRANOL

Dithranol (also called anthralin) is a complex organic substance that was originally obtained from natural sources but is now synthesized.

Conditions suited to treatment

Dithranol remains the most effective remedy for psoriasis though we still don't know how it works. It is not suitable for psoriasis of the scalp or for lesions in the flexures or on the face, but is helpful for plaque-type psoriasis of other sites providing it can be tolerated. It is generally used in concentrations of from 0.05 to 2 per cent, but rarely – in hospital patients – it is employed at concentrations of up to 12 per cent. Traditionally it has been used in a thick paste (Lassar's paste) or white soft paraffin and applied daily. It is now more often the practice to apply dithranol in the morning or evening for 30 minutes to 1 hour only, prior to having a bath. This has come to be known as 'short contact therapy' and seems to be at least as effective as more traditional techniques.

Unwanted side-effects

Dithranol should be used with care as it can irritate the skin of some patients quite badly; it is not known why these individuals are irritated and others are not. It used to be common-place to start off hospital in-patients with a very low concentration and slowly build up to the maximally tolerated concentration over a period of some two or three weeks. This practice is changing somewhat because the newer proprietary preparations that have become available in recent years – eg, Dithrocream, Dithrolan, Exolan, Psoradate, Stie-Lasan and anthralin stick (Anthraderm) – have made it suitable for routine use outside hospital.

Dithranol also stains the skin (and bedclothes) an unattractive and somewhat incon-venient brown-violet colour. Regrettably this seems to be a feature of all currently avail-able formulations.

SALICYLIC ACID

This is one of the oldest and most effective topical treatments in dermatology. It seems to work by 'unsticking' stratum corneum and aiding desquamation whenever there is scaling or hyperkeratosis.

Conditions suited to treatment

Salicylic acid is used in conditions as varied as the congenital ichthyoses, psoriasis, chronic dermatitic states, callosities and viral warts. It is contained in a vast number of preparations in concentrations of from 1 to 20 per cent, in vehicles ranging from ointments and gels to rapidly drying paints and occlusive films. It is particularly useful in a lotion of flexible collodion film in the treatment of warts. Two per cent salicylic acid ointment is of great help in treating hyperkeratotic and fissured dermatitis or psoriasis of the palms and soles. A 6 per cent preparation in propylene glycol gel is very effective in removing hyperkeratotic areas in very thick psoriasis and congenital disorders of keratinization.

Unwanted side-effects

Generally salicylic acid is not associated with serious side-effects but if large body areas are to be treated, enough can be absorbed through the skin to cause salicylism (as from taking too many aspirins).

SULPHUR

Sulphur preparations have been used for acne, rosacea, seborrhoeic dermatitis and scabies. There are now few real indications for their use. Sulphur seems to help get rid of scale in seborrhoeic dermatitis of the scalp and is still used in some proprietary preparations to help loosen blackheads in acne.

PRACTICAL POINTS

Preparation	Uses	Disadvantages	
Tar	● Psoriasis (particularly thick patches) ● Chronic dermatitic rashes	● Skin irritation ● Folliculitis ● Staining	● Smell ● Unpleasant appearance
Dithranol	● Plaque-type psoriasis	● Skin irritation	● Staining
Salicylic acid	● Congenital ichthyoses ● Psoriasis ● Chronic dermatitis ● Callosities ● Viral warts	● Irritation in higher concentrations ● Salicylism (rare)	
Sulphur	● Seborrhoeic dermatitis ● Acne	● Irritation in some individuals	

30

Prescribing hints for topical preparations

LOTION, GEL, OINTMENT, CREAM OR PASTE?

A great deal of fuss was made about the choice of vehicle for particular rashes in the dermatological practice of yesteryear. Generally speaking it is now realized that the particular vehicle is of less importance than what it contains; although this is not completely true as some of the vehicles seem to have therapeutic properties themselves! This is especially so of those that contain white soft paraffin, which have quite marked anti-inflammatory effects.

Acute rashes are best treated with either lotions or creams, while more chronic scaling rashes do best with ointments. Pastes are not too popular now, and there does not seem to be any special reason for prescribing them. Gels are less satisfactory than they might appear. Some seem to irritate and sting and are not well accepted by patients. Others are of course satisfactory and there is a place for them in the treatment of acne where some slight irritant effect could be an advantage.

Modern pharmaceutical formulation has succeeded in producing topical products that are cosmetically acceptable (and therefore will be used), nontoxic (and therefore do not irritate or sensitize), and deliver effectively their contained medicaments to the affected area. It should be noted that many modern topical agents are neither a cream nor an ointment but somewhere in between.

HOW MUCH TO PRESCRIBE

Practitioners frequently find it difficult to know exactly how much of an ointment or cream to give a patient. Clearly it depends on how long it is planned to continue the treatment and how large an area is affected by the disease. It is hard to give accurate guidelines but about 30 g of a material is necessary to cover an adult with an ointment on one occasion. Thus for someone with psoriasis who has about four large patches (about 100 cm^2 in total) and who will not be seen again for four weeks, about 50 g should suffice. For an atopic patient with widespread dermatitis 200 g may not be enough for a two-week period, and a watchful eye must be kept on the adequacy of the amount supplied.

Recently the idea of the 'fingertip unit' has been developed. This unit described the amount of cream or ointment that can be squeezed from a tube with a 5 mm nozzle to run between the index fingertip and the distal skin crease. The face and neck require 2.5 fingertip units and the front of the trunk needs 6.7 units.

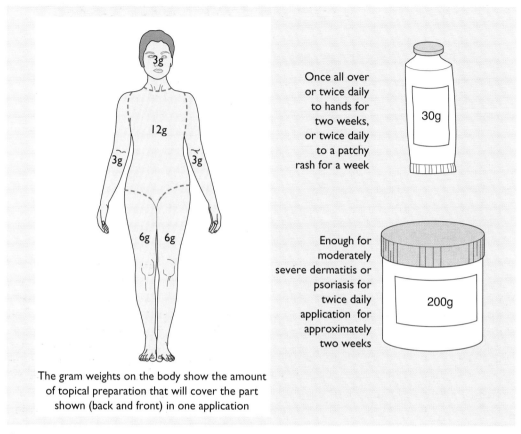

Once all over or twice daily to hands for two weeks, or twice daily to a patchy rash for a week

30g

Enough for moderately severe dermatitis or psoriasis for twice daily application for approximately two weeks

200g

The gram weights on the body show the amount of topical preparation that will cover the part shown (back and front) in one application

The gram weights on the body show the amount of topical preparation that will cover the part shown (back and front) in one application.

It is worth remembering that only the material in contact with the skin can do any good, and that only a thin smear is required. Creams usually spread better than ointments, so slightly less of these are required.

PRACTICAL POINTS

- White soft paraffin seems to have its own anti-inflammatory activity.
- Acute rashes are best treated with lotions or creams.
- Chronic scaling rashes respond better to ointments.
- 30 g of a topical medicament will cover an adult once.
- A thin smear is all that's necessary.

31

Diagnosis of scaling rashes

BACKGROUND

Scaliness of the skin's surface signifies that the process of horn formation is disturbed. The disturbance can be the result of an intrinsic abnormality of epidermal differentiation, as in congenital ichthyosis, or the result of inflammation, as in psoriasis and dermatitis. The accumulation of horn at a site has a similar significance to scaling – both represent the failure of the normal loss of horn cells at the surface as single cells.

Many scaling rashes are also red; if there is no redness and the scaling has been present since early childhood the diagnosis is probably that of ichthyosis. Occasionally a dry generalized scaling of the skin starts in later life and then there is a possibility of serious underlying disease, including neoplasia. Mild dryness and slight scaling (xeroderma) can also be caused by overenthusiastic bathing and dry cold weather, especially if the patient also has central heating at home.

Differentiating dermatitis and psoriasis

Appearance	Psoriasis has a distinct border and is raised up from the surface of normal skin, whereas dermatitic areas have less distinct margins and are not usually so raised.
Sites affected	Psoriasis preferentially involves the knees, elbows, sacrum and scalp. Atopic dermatitis preferentially affects the flexures but can involve any area. The other varieties of dermatitis can also have a characteristic distribution.
Symptoms	Dermatitis is characteristically itchy, but psoriasis does not usually irritate.
Family history	Both psoriasis and atopic dermatitis occur more frequently in families where one or other parent has the disorder. The other forms of dermatitis do not appear to run in families.
Natural history	Psoriasis is a lifelong remittent disorder; atopic dermatitis tends to improve with age. The other forms of dermatitis tend to be episodic and may only last for one attack.

GENERALIZED RED-SCALING RASHES

Psoriasis and dermatitis

These conditions are not usually difficult to distinguish from each other but even the expert can be foxed on occasions. Plaques of psoriasis almost always have a well-defined edge and a stuck-on-like appearance. The lesions are usually a beefy red and the surface covered with a crumbling silvery scale. The borders of large psoriatic patches are often 'festooned', in other words, seem to be composed of a series of semicircles because of the coalescence of a number of lesions. Psoriasis can occur anywhere on the skin but is particularly likely to affect the knees, elbows, scalp and back.

Dermatitis rashes vary in appearance according to the cause of the dermatitis and the stage the disease has reached. In general, dermatitic disorders are itchier than psoriasis and the results of scratching are more frequently seen. Recent scratches appear as irregularly interrupted linear erosions which become blood crusts. If scratching continues for long periods skin hypertrophy appears in which the affected area thickens and the superficial skin markings become accentuated. This process is known as lichenification and can occur in isolated well-defined patches looking a bit like psoriasis; this type of dermatitis goes by the name of circumscribed neurodermatitis or lichen simplex chronicus.

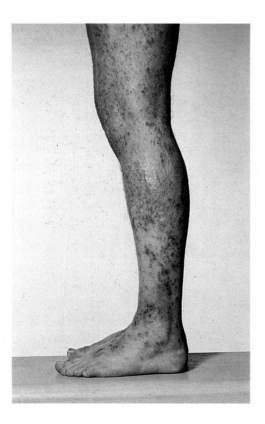

Severe atopic dermatitis affecting the legs.

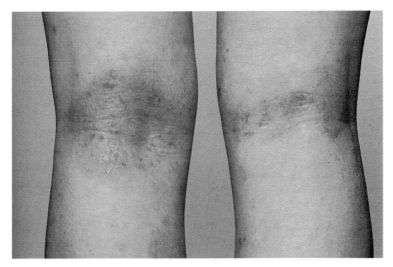

Lichenified atopic dermatitis affecting the popliteal fossae. This is a very characteristic site of involvement in this disease.

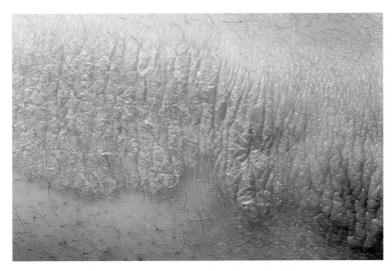

A well-defined thickened patch on which the skin markings are exaggerated. This condition is very itchy and known as lichen simplex chronicus or circumscribed neurodermatitis.

Confusingly, some patches of psoriasis can become dermatitic if they are persistently scratched. Another source of confusion may be seborrhoeic dermatitis on the front of the chest, face and scalp. This can look very much like psoriasis; indeed some dermatological wits have dubbed this 'seborrhiasis'.

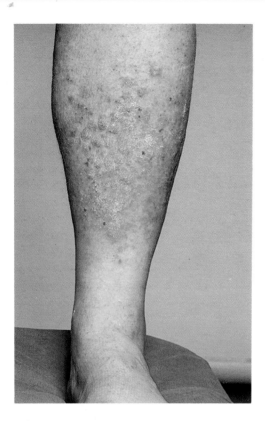

This man has long-standing psoriasis that is quite typical elsewhere. On the lower legs he finds it irritable and rubs and scratches it. The result is that it has a dermatitic, lichenified appearance.

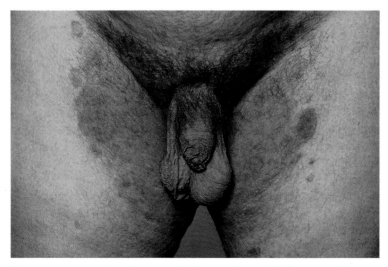

Ringworm of the groins (tinea cruris). The edge is well defined and although it affects both thighs it is not completely symmetrical.

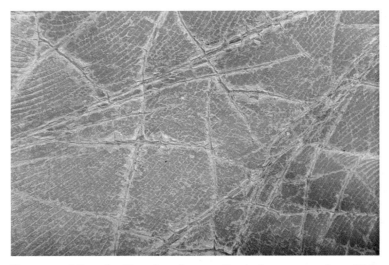

Ringworm of the palm. There is a silvery scaling in the creases and a reddish background to the skin.

Pityriasis rosea

This is a common scaling rash that mostly affects teenagers and young adults. A series of oval scaling macules appear on the trunk arranged characteristically along the lines of the ribs. The disorder usually lasts six to ten weeks.

Ringworm

This is usually easy to diagnose on the trunk. There is a sharp raised border with a tendency to clear inside the patch. On the trunk the lesion may be solitary or there may be two or three such areas. The diagnosis can be more difficult in the groin or on the hands and feet.

LOCALIZED RASHES

Scaling rashes in the groin

Flexural psoriasis of the groin is often misdiagnosed as ringworm or intertrigo. A history of recent onset, a spreading and well-defined, slightly redder and more raised edge and healing centre, and the absence of typical psoriasis elsewhere are in favour of ringworm. The only certain way of diagnosing ringworm is by taking a skin scraping for culture and direct microscopy for fungal micro-organisms. (In most localities a mycological laboratory will accept skin scrapings for examination.) The only certain way of confusing the issue and ultimately making the patient worse is by giving corticosteroids before a diagnosis has been established (see Chapter 27).

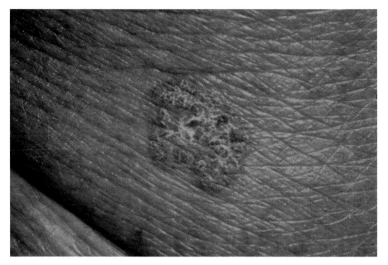

This well-defined scaling plaque looks psoriasiform but is in fact an area of Bowen's disease.

Intertrigo tends to affect areas of skin that rub together, so that the rash appears symmetrical. It also tends to spread to involve the apex of the groin whereas ringworm and psoriasis tend to be asymmetrical on either thigh and do not affect the apex of the groins.

Dermatitic rashes may also affect the groin but are usually part of a wider process, and there is evidence of rash elsewhere. Dermatitis rashes and intertrigo have an ill-defined border and may have excoriations on their surface or be lichenified.

Differential diagnosis of scaling rashes in the groin

- Ringworm
- Intertrigo
- Dermatitis
- Flexural psoriasis

Scaling rashes of the palms

When the palms are affected by a persistent scaling rash it may require a cluster of wise dermatologists to identify the cause. However, even the relative novice can be right much of the time if notice is taken of what follows. Let us assume that nowhere else is affected apart from the palms.

Dermatitic rashes There is often evidence of microvesiculation, that is, tiny little pin-prick marks on the surface due to oedema fluid breaking out. Cracks and fissures occur in both psoriasis and dermatitis but tend to be more frequent, with less tendency to heal, in chronic dermatitic rashes. The edges of palmar dermatitic rashes tend to be indistinct.

Psoriasis When the rash occurs in discrete patches on the palmar skin it is more likely to be due to psoriasis. Of course the history and the presence of rash elsewhere may be important in reaching a diagnostic conclusion.

Ringworm This usually affects one of the palms, although occasionally both may be affected. It causes a thin silvery scale on the surface, which tends to accumulate in the creases. Examination of the skin scales for fungal micro-organisms is important and may need to be repeated on several occasions.

Tests Many dermatologists (including the author) take the view that the clinical diagnosis of palmar rashes can be so difficult that skin scrapings should always be taken for fungus examination and patch tests arranged to see if allergic contact hypersensitivities are present. Even then, a biopsy may be required to help establish the cause (see Chapter 38).

Solitary scaling plaques

Psoriasis doesn't often affect just one body site for any protracted period; usually the patch is joined by others or it resolves.

Circumscribed neurodermatitis can remain at one site for long periods – on the ankle, the sacrum, the forearm or the back of the scalp and neck, for example. It usually bears the hallmark of constant scratching.

Intraepidermal epithelioma (Bowen's disease) can present as a solitary 'psoriasis-like' patch on the arms, legs or trunk (see page 157). Scaling round red plaques on the front

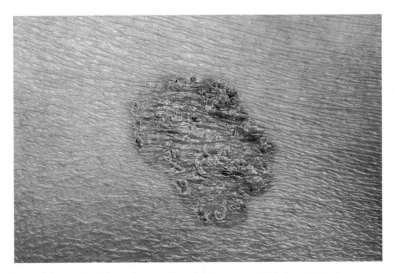

Superficial basal cell carcinoma. The edge is very well defined and close inspection shows that it is slightly raised and pearly.

Solitary scaling plaques

- Psoriasis
- Circumscribed neurodermatitis
- Ringworm
- Bowen's disease
- Solar keratoses
- Superficial basal cell epithelioma

of the lower legs in middle-aged and elderly women often turn out to be patches of Bowen's disease.

Solar keratoses are usually smaller but can present in the same way as Bowen's disease.

Occasionally a superficial basal cell epithelioma will present as a solitary scaling patch. However, this disorder, which mostly affects the upper trunk, is usually characterized by a very distinctive, slightly raised, thin hair-like margin.

LESS COMMON CAUSES OF SCALING

Lichen planus

This is a not uncommon itchy papular rash that occasionally gives rise to scaling plaques. On the palms and soles it can look very much like dermatitis or psoriasis. On the limbs it can be difficult to distinguish from circumscribed neurodermatitis. The

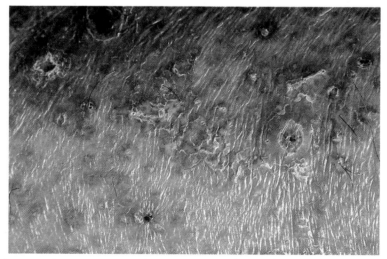

Lichen planus. The papules in this disease are small, polygonal and flat topped and have a mauve tint.

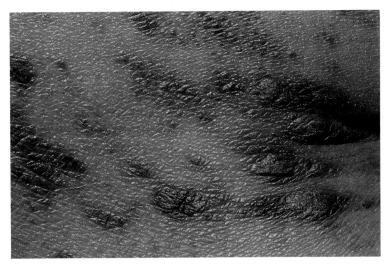

Lichen planus of the trunk. There are papules and pigmentation from previous lesions. The pigmentation is typical of healing areas.

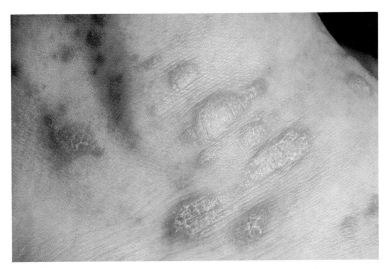

This patient also has lichen planus. There is a slight scale to the lesions. Some of the smaller papules have coalesced to form plaques. Closer inspection of some of the lesions shows whitish lines known as Wickham's striae.

papular rash has a typical mauve colouration and this may be a useful distinguishing feature even when the papules have coalesced into a scaling plaque. Close inspection will often reveal faint white lines in the substance of the papule. These are known as Wickham's striae.

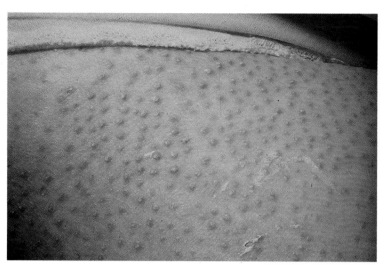

Pityriasis rubra pilaris. In this condition each follicle mouth is raised, red or pink and scaling in some areas.

Mycosis fungoides

This is a malignant T-cell lymphoma affecting the skin. It starts off with psoriasiform or dermatitic-looking patches on the trunk and then progresses. If the scaling areas stay in one place for long periods and then gradually extend and thicken, suspicions should be aroused. Fortunately it is rare.

Pityriasis rubra pilaris

This is a rare scaling disorder that looks like psoriasis on some occasions and very distinctive on others. Typically it tends to affect hair follicles particularly so that horny spines are evident in some sites. It also has a typical orangey colour – particularly on the palms. The face and scalp are usually involved early on in the disease. It tends to last on average about 2 years.

PRACTICAL POINTS

- Scaling with no redness since early childhood is probably a form of ichthyosis.
- Be alert to the possibility of serious underlying disease if generalized dry scaly skin starts later in life.
- Psoriatic lesions are characterized by a well-defined edge, a red colour and a surface of crumbling silvery scales.
- Dermatitic disorders are usually itchier than psoriasis and scratch marks are a more frequent feature.
- Don't give corticosteroids for scaling rashes in the groin until diagnosis has been established.

32

Diagnosis of acute and generalized rashes

BACKGROUND

One of the commonest diagnostic problems for the practitioner, as far as skin disorders are concerned, is a generalized rash that arises quite unexpectedly over a day or two. In most instances the problem is easily solved if a few simple hints are remembered.

RASHES DUE TO INFECTIOUS FEVERS

The first step is to establish whether the rash is part of an infectious fever or whether there is some other cause. Rashes due to infectious fevers are usually preceded by some form of general unwellness with sore throat, fever and aches and pains. This is not invariable, though, and young, otherwise fit adults may not notice much else apart from the rash. An important clue is a history of contact with someone else with the disorder or at least a person who was incubating it at the time of contact. Eruptions due to infectious fever consist in most cases of flat red spots (macules) or spots that are slightly raised (maculopapules). These are not usually markedly elevated (like a boil or insect bite) and when they first appear are not often scaly (like psoriasis).

Measles and German measles

Measles is not usually confused with anything else, but German measles (rubella) can be difficult to distinguish. Enlargement of posterior auricular lymph nodes may help identify youngsters with German measles. It goes without saying that German measles sufferers should be kept away from pregnant women.

Glandular fever

A generalized macular or maculopapular rash can develop in glandular fever. Interestingly, when ampicillin is given in glandular fever in the mistaken belief that the sore throat is due to bacterial infection it seems to precipitate the rash. It is then not certain whether the rash is due to the drug, the complaint or a combination of both.

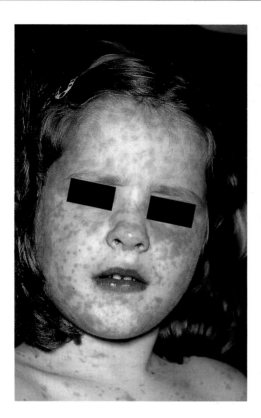

This little girl has measles. There is a macular erythematous rash affecting the entire trunk.

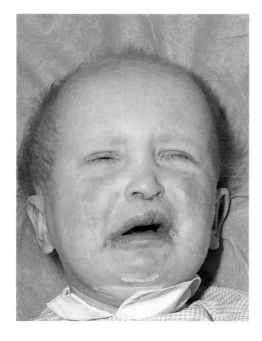

Measles. This youngster is clearly miserable. There is soreness and crusting around the lips and eyes, and a degree of photophobia from conjunctivitis of the eyes. There is also some reddening of the cheeks and forehead.

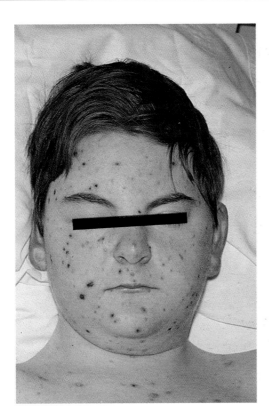

Chickenpox. Typical crusted vesicles can be seen on this young man's face.

Chickenpox

Chickenpox usually presents as generalized papular and vesicular rash. The individual spots tend to be concentrated on the upper trunk, face and upper limbs but can occur elsewhere. It is not usually confused with anything else.

Roseola infantum

Like other infectious diseases of childhood, roseola infantum is quite mild with only slight unwellness. There is a rash that lasts some two to four days only.

Secondary syphilis

The rash of secondary syphilis can be difficult to recognize and it is only by being aware of the possibility of the disease that mistakes can be avoided. It can be papular, or psoriasis-like, or macular and German measles-like. There is usually some mild feeling of unwellness and even some fever. Important clues are to be found in the mouth, where there are erosions, and perianally, where warty lesions (condyloma lata) are to be found (see page 132). There is often lymph node enlargement in the neck, axillae and groins. The rash tends to persist and is not generally very itchy. Of course the history of a genital

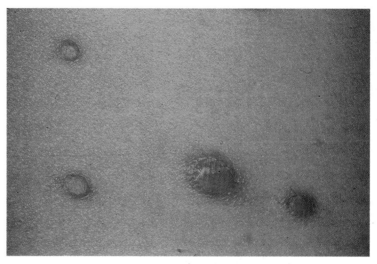

Papular lesions on the trunk in a patient with secondary syphilis.

sore in the recent past is enormously helpful but unfortunately not always forthcoming. If there is any suspicion that secondary syphilis is the cause of the patient's rash he or she should be seen by a specialist as an urgent case.

HIV infection

A generalized erythematous maculopapular rash with mild fever and malaise without particular features may be seen in some patients a few weeks after being infected with the human immunodeficiency virus (HIV) and about the time they become 'antigen positive'.

RASHES DUE TO OTHER CAUSES

If there is no fever, no systemic upset and no history of contact with someone with a similar complaint it is unlikely that an infectious fever is the cause.

Drugs

Drug-induced rashes (see also Chapter 13) may sometimes mimic infectious illnesses but close attention to the history should enable the distinction to be made. Fever and malaise may accompany the onset of a drug reaction, with a dramatically sudden onset of a generalized rash. The type of eruption that develops depends on a variety of factors but predominantly on the nature of the drug responsible.

Urticarial rashes These are most often caused by penicillin and related antibiotics, salicylates, morphine alkaloids and blood products.

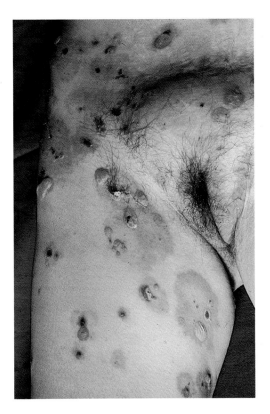

This elderly woman developed red urticaria-like patches over her trunk quite suddenly. Many of the areas became blistered. Histology and immunofluorescence tests confirmed the clinical suspicion that she had pemphigoid.

Morbilliform (measles-like) maculopapular rashes These are produced by antirheumatic drugs, antibiotics (ampicillin in particular), diuretics and psychotropic agents and can be difficult to distinguish from real measles.

Acute generalized rashes The most serious are those that blister and erode the skin. Severe erythema multiforme (Stevens–Johnson syndrome) and toxic epidermal necrolysis are in this category. These are usually easy to distinguish from other acute rashes because of the accompanying systemic disturbance and the blistering and/or erosive nature of the skin disorder. They may be caused by anti-inflammatory and antithyroid drugs, diuretics, gold injections and oral hypoglycaemics.

Rare blistering diseases

Patients with the rare blistering diseases pemphigus, pemphigoid and dermatitis herpetiformis (see Chapter 35) usually develop their respective skin lesions over a few days or even a few weeks (though pemphigoid can have an acute onset) and the onset is not often accompanied by fever or malaise.

Purpuric rashes

Rashes with a purpuric element require particular care as they may indicate a severe underlying disease such as leukaemia or thrombocytopenic purpura. If the spots are raised up and there are also areas that look urticarial, the condition is more likely to be Henoch–Schönlein purpura (allergic vasculitis). Abdominal pain, arthritis and fever may accompany this type of rash. If purpura is present in the rash, pressure on the spots will not blanch the redness.

Psoriasis

Psoriasis (see also Chapters 19 and 31) can break out quite dramatically over a day or two, even if there has been no previous history of the disorder. Three types may be generalized and acute.

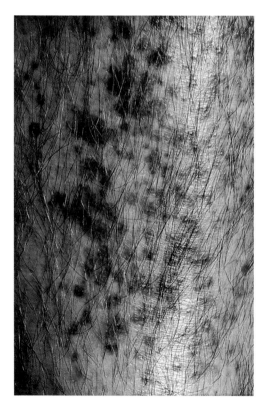

Anaphylactoid purpura in an elderly man who also had glomerulonephritis as a result of his disease.

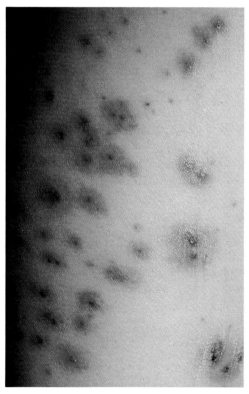

Anaphylactoid purpura (Henoch-Schönlein syndrome). Over the space of a day or two this young man developed urticarial areas, some of which were purpuric. His joints also became painful and he had abdominal pain.

Guttate psoriasis This usually occurs in children and young adults up to the age of about 15 or 16 and often follows an episode of streptococcal tonsillitis. The spots in this type of psoriasis are small and not as scaly as in ordinary plaque-type psoriasis. They are spattered all over the trunk and limbs and are all at the same stage of development (see pages 17–18).

Erythrodermic psoriasis In adults, psoriasis can suddenly worsen to become erythrodermic, with the redness and scaling spreading all over the body. Patients with this complication can be extremely ill; luckily this is relatively rare. They lose heat and fluid through their damaged skin and need in-patient care in a unit familiar with the problems involved.

Pustular psoriasis This can be persistent and localized to the palms and soles, or it can be generalized. The generalized variety, which goes by the eponym Von Zumbusch's disease, is a rare and most unpleasant disorder. It starts abruptly with showers of tiny pus spots (pustules) appearing on skin that may or may not show generalized redness. There is usually considerable systemic disturbance and often a fever which precedes the pustules. As with erythrodermic psoriasis, patients with generalized pustular psoriasis urgently need expert care and attention.

Dermatitis

Dermatitic rashes can also suddenly become generalized. The skin of some patients with atopic dermatitis (see also Chapter 15) seems curiously labile; one minute they are fine with only a few lichenified scaling patches and some generalized dryness, while the next the inflammation has spread all over the body and they are in acute discomfort. Unfortunately many such episodes are quite unpredictable.

Occasionally other types of dermatitis suddenly become generalized. The clue as far as dermatitis is concerned is the intense itching that accompanies the rash. Close examination of the skin may reveal the presence of numerous tiny water blisters (vesicles).

Lichen planus

Lichen planus is an itchy papular disorder of unknown cause that can appear all over the trunk and limbs within a few days (see page 191). The individual spots have a mauve colour and tend to be flat-topped. In about half the patients the buccal mucosa becomes involved with a white lacework or white dot pattern.

Pityriasis rosea

This is a fairly common disorder that doesn't seem to cause too much of a problem in diagnosis. It mostly affects young adults or teenagers. Often the patient reports that one large patch first appeared on the trunk ('herald patch') to be followed three or four days later by a generalized eruption of oval scaly pink patches (macules). Each spot is 2 cm or more in diameter and they tend to be arranged around the trunk so that the long axes of the macules follow the lines of the ribs.

PRACTICAL POINTS

- Rashes due to infectious fevers are often preceded by sore throat, fever and aches and pains, and contact with someone with a similar complaint.
- The rash of secondary syphilis is usually accompanied by oral erosions and sometimes by perianal condyloma lata.
- Drugs that can cause acute generalized rashes include:
  –Antibiotics (especially ampicillin and penicillin)
  –Anti-inflammatory drugs
  –Antirheumatics
  –Antithyroid drugs
  –Diuretics
  –Gold injections
  –Oral hypoglycaemics
  –Psychotropics.
- Purpuric rashes may indicate severe underlying systemic disease. Pressure on the spots of purpuric rashes will not blanch the redness.
- Patients with erythrodermic and generalized pustular psoriasis need urgent specialist care.

33

Diagnosis of rashes on the face

BACKGROUND

Facial skin is thinner and more delicate than skin elsewhere and unlike most other areas has numerous densely packed large hair follicles and sebaceous glands. It also has a very distensible blood supply that reaches very near the surface. Two other features of facial skin set it aside from other areas – it is the area of skin most exposed to sunlight and airborne allergens and it is very important in social recognition and communication. All this may explain why some common rashes look different on the face while other skin disorders occur on facial skin alone.

DIAGNOSTIC POINTERS

Dermatitis and psoriasis

Atopic dermatitis Facial skin is often involved in atopic dermatitis and the resulting appearance is characteristic. The skin seems dry and finely scaling but the front and sides of the neck may show a rippling or reticular pattern of pigmentation. There is slight pallor of the facial skin and extra creases below the eyes. This atopic creasing is probably the result of oedema and thickening from continual rubbing of the eyes due to irritation.

Allergic contact dermatitis This often picks out the face either because the sensitizing agent is airborne in the environment or because the allergen has been inadvertently transferred there by the hands (see Chapter 34). The eyelids and sides of the neck are the sites that are usually involved.

Seborrhoeic dermatitis This is a common distinctive form of eczema now believed to be due to infection with pityrosporum ovale – a yeast-like micro-organism that commonly lives on normal skin. Its name is misleading because it is not due to disease of the sebaceous glands and those with the condition do not necessarily have a greasy skin. It is best thought of as a 'constitutional' disorder, being a persistent skin problem in predisposed individuals. Although there is a type of dermatitis in infants that is labelled 'seborrhoeic', this is probably not the same disease. Seborrhoeic dermatitis is essentially an adults' disease.

Characteristically, diffuse red scaling patches occur in the nasolabial grooves, in and behind the ears and on the scalp and eyebrows. The front of the chest and the major body

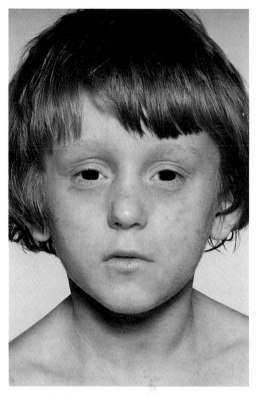

Typical atopic facies. Notice the comparative loss of eye lashes and slight swelling around the eyes with an extra crease.

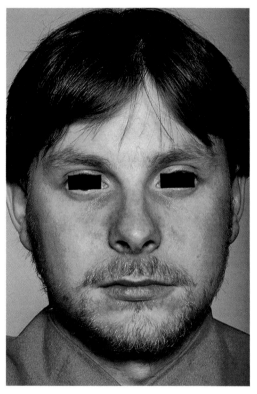

Mild seborrhoeic dermatitis affecting the face. Perinasal areas and the eyebrows are affected with a pink scaling rash.

flexures may also be affected. In the elderly the disorder may spread to affect large areas of skin and may even become erythrodermic. Seborrhoeic dermatitis tends to flare at times of stress and lasts for several weeks or months before subsiding for a variable period.

Perioral dermatitis This is a papular disorder of the face that is less common now than it used to be – probably because potent corticosteroids are less used on the face than they once were. This condition is distinguished by myriads of tiny papules occurring around the mouth, and responds quickly to oral tetracyline.

Psoriasis This does not often affect facial skin, and when it does it tends to look and behave like seborrhoeic dermatitis.

Rosacea and acne

Rosacea This is a common inflammatory disorder of facial skin of unknown cause. It affects more women than men, the highest incidence being in the fourth and fifth decades. It is characterized by persistent erythema of the cheeks and maybe the forehead, nose and chin as well. Rosacea only rarely affects the skin outside the face and neck. The

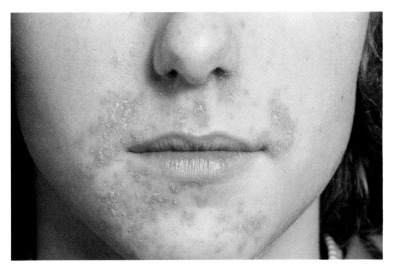

Numerous small pustules around the mouth are typical of perioral dermatitis.

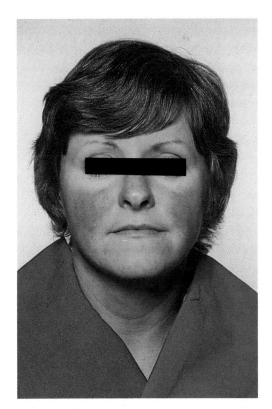

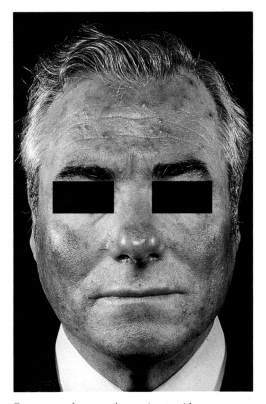

Symmetrically reddened cheeks in a patient with rosacea. Later she developed inflamed papules on the affected sites.

Rosacea made worse by corticosteroid creams.

Rosacea
- Most often affects 30- to 40-year-old women
- Erythema of cheeks, forehead, nose and chin
- Redness, telangiectasia and oedema are very common features

Acne
- Mostly affects teenagers. Men most severely affected
- Papules on face, neck, shoulders, back and chest
- Usually less red than rosacea

affected areas are also telangiectatic and generally brighter red than in acne; they may be somewhat oedematous. Episodically papules and pustules develop on the reddened areas. These differ from those in acne in that they are not tender, do not occur outside of the face and are unassociated with blackheads and seborrhoea. In addition cysts do not form as they may do in acne, and scarring does not result.

The response to treatment is quite different also. In rosacea there is usually a rapid response to orally administered tetracycline – that is, about 75 per cent of patients show great improvement in four to six weeks. The erythema in rosacea tends to be persistent, although there are recurrent acute episodes of papules and swelling which are short-lived.

Acne This affects both sexes equally although men tend to be more severely affected. It is usually a teenage disease but may drag on until the third and fourth decades. More uncommonly it affects older people and, rarely, may even affect infants.

Acne involves the shoulders, back and chest as well as the face and neck. Sometimes the skin on which the acne papules arise becomes reddened due to treatment or the damage caused by the disease and this redness is sometimes confused with rosacea.

PRACTICAL POINTS

- Many common skin diseases look different when they occur on the face.
- Diagnostic features of facial atopic dermatitis are:
  –Dry, finely scaling skin
  –Rippling pigmentation on neck
  –Facial pallor
  –Creasing below the eyes.
- Facial psoriasis is similar in appearance and behaviour to seborrhoeic dermatitis.
- In general, the use of steroid creams and ointments on facial skin is to be discouraged – especially the potent and very potent preparations – as they make rosacea, acne and perioral dermatitis worse (see Chapter 27).
- If some anti-inflammatory preparation is necessary, as in atopic dermatitis or occasionally in psoriasis, then hydrocortisone or other low-potency preparation should be used.

34

Allergy: urticaria and dermatitis

BACKGROUND

I find that the term allergy is very poorly understood by both the general public and medical students, and sometimes even by practitioners and dermatologists. Its original meaning was that of a specific acquired hypersensitivity but it later came to imply hypersensitivity of the immediate type. Unfortunately it has become firmly implanted in the mind of the public as indicating any type of adverse reaction to a foreign material. To avoid confusion it would probably be best to dispense with the term allergy altogether and use instead hypersensitivity with an appropriate qualifying adjective: immediate hypersensitivity or delayed hypersensitivity.

URTICARIA

Diagnosis

Urticaria is the typical skin response in immediate hypersensitivity. It is the sort of reaction seen after eating seafood such as lobster or soon after an injection of penicillin. The individual spots are itchy, raised, pink or red papules or larger swellings. Characteristically they come and go, and only remain at the same site for a few hours. Sometimes deeper, large, skin-coloured swellings are seen and these lesions are known as angio-oedema. When there is a very severe attack there may be associated systemic signs including wheezing, vomiting and/or abdominal pain and diarrhoea, and even hypotension and collapse.

Causes

Urticarial lesions do not result only from immediate hypersensitivity and this often makes it difficult to sort out the cause of a particular patient's urticaria. For example, small and quickly fading urticarial spots are quite common after a hot bath or after vigorous exercise. This condition is known as cholinergic urticaria.

Urticaria may also occur after intake of drugs (including aspirin and the morphine-type alkaloids) which provoke the release of histamine from mast cells. These drugs and some food additives can also aggravate or precipitate urticaria without actually being the underlying cause. Urticarial lesions may also sometimes be caused by physical stimuli, such as cold temperatures, pressure and solar irradiation.

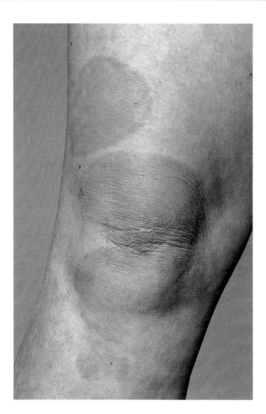

Urticarial patches in a young man.

Urticarial lesions are also a feature of some serious systemic disorders in which there is a complex immunological component, including anaphylactoid purpura and lupus erythematosus.

Management

It is slightly easier to pinpoint a cause of urticaria when it is of recent onset than when it has been present for many months. Even then, my guess is that we are lucky if we can nail down the cause in 10 per cent of patients. Nonetheless, I believe that an attempt should be made to exclude the common known causes of urticaria and to identify those factors that make it worse in the rest. Specialist prick or scratch testing is one appropriate procedure, but other more sophisticated tests may be required (see Chapter 38). Investigation will determine those sufferers who have a food allergy or whose condition is made worse by a constituent of food. Complex exclusion diets may help these patients, but will give no help to the remainder.

Some patients seem to be helped by antihistamines; others are not. In the latter group a few respond well to a combination of one of the conventional antihistamines (H_1 antagonists) with one of the H_2 antagonists, eg, cimetidine (Tagamet).

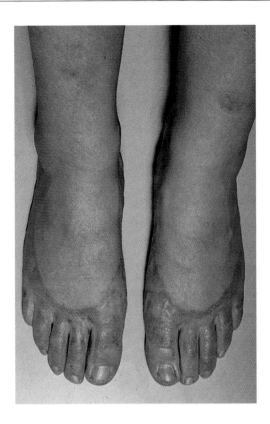

Allergic contact dermatitis due to sensitivity to a dye in the shoe material. Note the very characteristic distribution.

Papular urticaria

This condition is not really urticaria at all but a widespread papular reaction to insect bites. Some of the itchy spots seem to have identifiable bites or puncture marks on their surface while others do not. These spots are less evanescent and more uniform in appearance than ordinary urticaria.

DERMATITIS

As mentioned previously, dermatitis and eczema are synonyms for a common type of inflammation of the skin. Some types appear to be due to as yet unidentified constitutional abnormalities while others are more obviously the result of some external set of circumstances. Allergic contact dermatitis is the only member of this group of disorders in which hypersensitivity is known to be to blame. The hypersensitivity is of the delayed type and is lymphocyte-mediated.

The most frequent type of allergic contact dermatitis is nickel dermatitis. In this disease a dermatitic rash breaks out at the site of contact with nickel-containing articles such as clips on underclothes or inexpensive jewellery. It seems that the nickel in the metal of

Some common causes of allergic contact dermatitis (ACD)

Metals	Nickel is an extremely common cause. Around 5 per cent or even more of the female population is sensitive to nickel but it is only responsible for dermatitis in a few of these. Nickel may be found in jewellery, clips, fasteners, handles and coins. Nickel-sensitive individuals may also be sensitive to chromates, which may be found in some cements and are occasionally used to tan leather (eg, cause of shoe dermatitis). Silver and gold very rarely cause ACD
Flowers, fruit and vegetables	Primulae and chrysanthemums. In the United States, poison ivy. Some woods (eg, rose wood). Various citrus fruit extracts, eg, extracts of orange, lemon and Bergamot. Onions and garlic. In Australia, the Japanese wax tree
Chemicals, plastics, adhesives and dyes	Formaldehyde and formaldehyde resins, epoxy glues, rubber additives (eg, mercaptobenzthiazole), paraphenylenediamine and similar dyes (used as hair dyes), various additives to plastics
Materials used in creams and ointments, and cosmetics	Lanoline, neomycin, sulphanomides, penicillin, cinchocaine, amethocaine, some antihistamines, parabenz compounds, balsam of Peru, perfumes, emulsifying agents and other additives

the clip or jewellery is leached out and joins on to some protein in the epidermis. It is this protein–nickel complex to which the hypersensitivity arises. Other common sensitizers appear in the table above.

Diagnosis and management

There are several important points to be remembered for successful diagnosis and management of allergic contact dermatitis.

Identifying the sensitizer The rash occurs mainly at the sites of contact although it may take some good detective work to find out how a particular anatomical site comes to be involved. Dermatitis of the left thigh, the hands and eyelids in a member of our hospital staff turned out to be due to one of the constituents of 'strike-anywhere' matches. He was a pipe smoker and kept the matches in his left-hand trouser pocket – his eyelids had been affected by the fumes! Dermatitis of the right upper arm and antecubital fossa in a young medical student turned out to be due to a sensitivity to a constituent of one of his girlfriend's cosmetic creams which contacted his arm when she slept on it.

Superadded hypersensitivity The connection between the sensitizer and the sensitized may not always be as contorted as the examples I have quoted but it is easy to be caught out.

Although a dermatitis may not initially be due to hypersensitivity, allergic contact dermatitis may become superimposed on it. This is the case in those unlucky patients who develop sensitivity to a constituent of one of the creams or ointments used to treat them. Neomycin, lanolin, local anaesthetics and antihistamines are among the many substances that can cause this type of problem. It is even possible to become sensitized to corticosteroids in topical corticosteroid preparations. Patients with gravitational eczema seem particularly liable to develop this type of secondary contact hypersensitivity (see Chapter 23).

Patch testing Even when the pattern of the dermatitis appears unlikely to be due to contact hypersensitivity, patch tests should be performed (see Chapter 38). These are best carried out in specialist departments as there are many traps to ensnare the inexperienced. Essentially the test involves placing the suspected material(s) in close contact with the skin over a 48-hour period and then inspecting the site subsequently for the development of a dermatitic patch at the site of application. Usually a battery of substances is put on the skin at one time. The ones chosen are those with which the patient is most likely to have come into contact, and may also contain substances known to be common contact sensitizers in the community – rubber chemicals and black dye, for instance. Patch testing has become a complex investigation and some dermatology departments run special patch test and other investigative clinics for occupational dermatitis.

Very minute quantities of the sensitizer may be enough to set off the reaction in someone who is very sensitive. I have known patients who merely had to sniff at a primula before breaking out in dermatitis. Other sensitized individuals may develop their rash merely by walking into a factory containing the particular adhesive or rubber additive to which they react.

Management Corticosteroids may be used to treat an acute contact dermatitis rash, but as the condition is self-limiting they may not be required if the sensitizer is identified and the patient avoids contact with it. To help prevent recurrence, every effort should be made to avoid contact with any materials to which the patient is known to be sensitized. This, of course, may lead to problems at work (see Chapter 6).

PRACTICAL POINTS

Urticaria

- Common sensitizers include penicillin and seafood.
- Urticaria may also be precipitated by:
  - Aspirin
  - Morphine-type alkaloids
  - Hot baths
  - Exercise
  - The cold
  - Pressure
  - Sun exposure.
- Urticaria may rarely point to a systemic disorder.
- Management:
  1. Attempt to identify sensitizer and agents that aggravate the condition.
  2. If it is a food, try eliminating it from the diet.
  3. Prescribe antihistamines (H_1 antagonists) – if unsuccessful add an H_2 antagonist.

Allergic contact dermatitis

- A very common cause is nickel, which is found in a wide variety of everyday and household items.
- Detailed questioning of the patient may be needed to identify the sensitizer.
- Gravitational dermatitis sufferers often develop allergic contact dermatitis caused by constituents of the creams and ointments used to treat them.
- Specialist patch testing is essential for accurate diagnosis.

35

Diagnosis of skin diseases that blister

BACKGROUND

Blisters occur in many skin disorders, and it takes a practised eye to diagnose them correctly. They are especially difficult to identify at the start of the illness as their appearance may be quite untypical. Some diseases blister occasionally or only at one stage of their course. Others are primarily blistering and blister from the beginning of the disorder.

The skin is composed of tissues that are tightly bonded together and when a blister forms it signifies that the structure has been seriously disturbed, with individual elements falling apart. In general, the primary blistering disorders are quite serious, and when blistering occurs in the course of a normally nonblistering disease it signifies that the disease has adopted a more aggressive pattern.

Blistering can occur from damage to the tissues at the junction between the epidermis and the dermis or it can occur because the epidermal cells fall apart so that fluid accumulates between them.

THE BLISTERING SKIN DISEASES

No other group of skin diseases has been so intensively studied in recent years, and understanding of their nature and the processes involved has advanced tremendously. One consequence has been the development of good diagnostic tests for those blistering diseases that are immunologically based. Detailed descriptions of the individual blistering diseases would be out of place in this book. Although fascinating, they are uncommon; the general practitioner may expect to encounter such a problem only once every 2 or 3 years. They nonetheless deserve mention here because of the problems that arise from misdiagnosis.

Pemphigus

This is a disease of adults of any age and either sex. It usually begins with one or two eroded areas, often in the flexures. The mouth is frequently involved, with unpleasantly eroded areas. The lesions increase in size and number until large areas of skin are involved and the patient becomes quite ill. The individual lesions are either flaccid, thin-walled blisters or sloughy erosions due to the blisters forming within the epidermis.

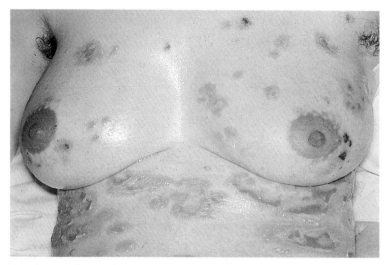

Pemphigus vulgaris. This patient has many erosions and flaccid blistered areas of the skin of the trunk. The condition developed quite suddenly. Histological examination and immunofluorescence tests confirmed the fact that she had pemphigus.

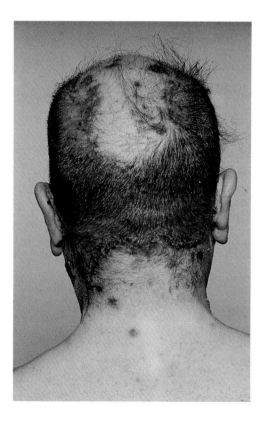

This elderly man also had a form of pemphigus. The onset was quite insidious. The mouth was extensively involved as well as the skin.

Senile pemphigoid

As the name suggests, this mainly affects the elderly. The blisters may appear explosively and affect many body sites. They are tense and, because they form subepidermally, tend to contain blood-stained fluid.

Dermatitis herpetiformis

This persistent itchy blistering rash occurs initially on the buttocks, elbows, knees and scalp but can occur anywhere. There are also red urticarial-like patches on which the blisters may arise. The blisters tend to be small and grouped together (herpetiform vesicles).

Epidermolysis bullosa

This is the name for a group of congenital blistering disorders in which there are faults in the way the epidermis and dermis are joined together. In the most severe forms it can result in the most ghastly scarring and deformity. I have seen it misdiagnosed as staphylococcal infection of the newborn – which can also blister. It is important to reach a diagnosis quickly to avoid unnecessary treatment and to inform the parents about the prognosis as soon as possible.

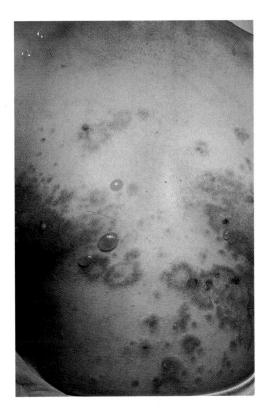

Dermatitis herpetiformis. There are many reddened areas, some of which have blisters in them. Apart from the trunk, this man's itchy rash affected the knees, elbows and scalp. It was controlled quite easily with dapsone by mouth.

The blisters and erosions occur on the fingers, hands and feet, buttocks and in the mouth mainly – as they arise primarily at sites of trauma. The surrounding skin is not inflamed and there are few other distinguishing features.

Accurate characterization may require sophisticated tests, and specialist units with experience with this disease should be consulted.

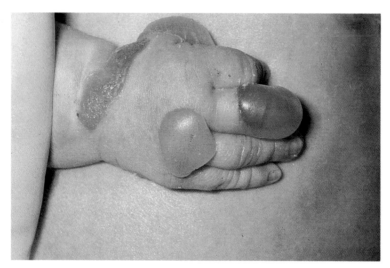

Dystrophic epidermolysis bullosa. Large tense blisters have occurred at the peripheral sites in this young child. The mouth was also extensively involved, making feeding difficult.

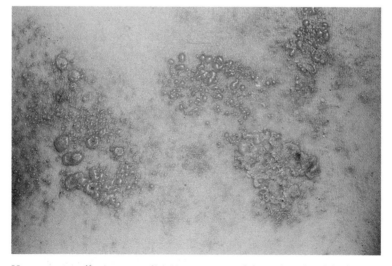

Herpes zoster affecting two adjoining segments of the right side of the lower chest wall in an elderly woman. The affected areas were painful and hyperaesthetic. There were many small vesicles clustered together in the involved areas which later became crusted and exudative.

Porphyria cutanea tarda

This is a serious metabolic disorder in which there is marked photosensitivity. On exposed areas the skin may blister and become pigmented. Curious hypertrichosis can occur on the face. There is usually underlying liver disease. Diagnosis is reached by finding abnormal porphyrin excretion in the stools and urine.

OTHER DISORDERS OF THE SKIN THAT MAY CAUSE VESICULATION OR BLISTERING

Chickenpox

Chickenpox vesicles are usually easy to recognize (see page 195). Shingles (herpes zoster) is no more than chickenpox localized to the distribution of a dorsal sensory nerve root in someone who has had chickenpox previously, ie, it only occurs in 'immune' individuals.

Cold sores (herpes simplex)

These characteristically cause sore red patches on which vesicles develop around the mouth or nose recurrently. It is also quite often seen on the buttocks and around the genitalia (see Chapter 9).

Hand, foot and mouth disease

This is a mild viral infection in which vesicles occur on the palms and soles and sometimes the buttocks. Lesions are also seen inside the mouth.

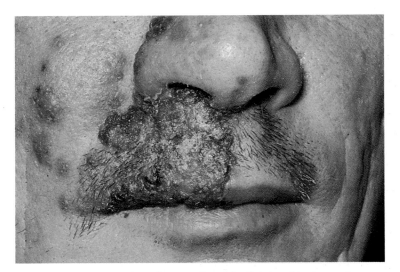

Herpes zoster affecting the right upper lip and adjoining skin due to the involvement of the maxillary branch of the fifth nerve. The condition is at a later stage than in the previous picture and shows considerable crusting.

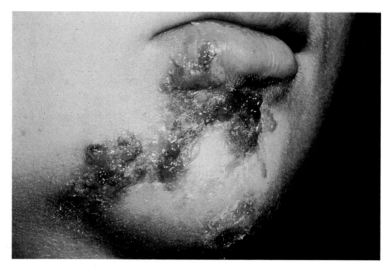

Extensive crusted herpes simplex affecting the lower lip in a child who had not experienced herpes simplex before (primary herpes simplex). There were areas of involvement inside the mouth and there was some slight fever and malaise.

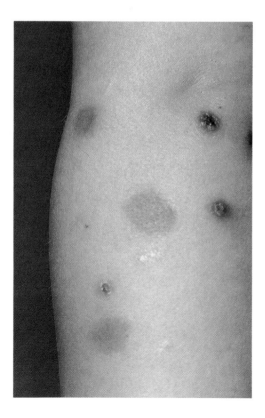

Insect bites on the legs of a young woman.

Impetigo

This is a bacterial infection of the skin which is mostly a disorder of young children, but can occur in other age groups too. The primary lesion is an oozy red crusted patch on the face or, less frequently, the trunk or limbs. Large blisters can also occur – especially, as mentioned previously, in newborn infants.

Scabies infestation

Not characteristically blistering, but vesicles sometimes occur around the wrist or fingers (see Chapter 25).

Insect bites

Don't be caught out by these! I have seen young, otherwise fit patients rushed to hospital with all kinds of exotic diagnoses, who had merely served as mobile meals for hordes of mosquitoes or midges. The bites of bedbugs and fleas can also blister.

Dermatitis

Dermatitis can and does blister sometimes. The basic problem in dermatitis is inflammation within the epidermis. If the inflammation is particularly vigorous and rapid in onset, vesicles or even quite large blisters can form. There is usually some evidence of dermatitis elsewhere and the affected areas are terribly itchy.

PRACTICAL POINTS

- Blistering disorders are rare but can be quite serious. They include:
  –Pemphigus
  –Senile pemphigoid
  –Erythema multiforme
  –Dermatitis herpetiformis
  –Epidermolysis bullosa
  –Porphyria cutanea tarda.
- When blistering occurs in a normally nonblistering disease it indicates that the disease has taken a more aggressive course. Other skin disorders that can blister include:
  –Chickenpox
  –Herpes simplex
  –Herpes zoster
  –Hand, foot and mouth disease
  –Impetigo
  –Insect bites
  –Dermatitis.

36

Diagnosis of moles, warts, nodules, cancers and cysts

BACKGROUND

The diagnosis of warty and nonwarty knobs, lumps and bumps of the skin appears to be much easier than it actually is. These lesions are extremely common and consultation for them constitutes an important aspect of practice. Because of their frequency and the potentially serious results of misdiagnosis we all need to improve our diagnostic skills in this area of medicine.

PIGMENTED LESIONS

Pigmented lesions present particular problems. Several studies have shown that even the most experienced dermatologist makes mistakes when it comes to differentiating the various pigmented lumps and bumps. Moles and seborrhoeic warts are the commonest

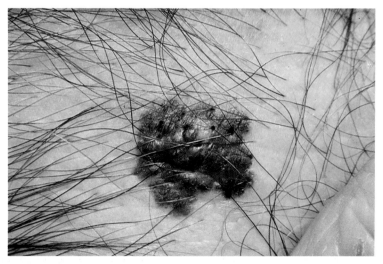

Malignant melanoma. A small, flat, brown area on the left side of the chest wall of this 50-year-old man had reached this size and appearance in a period of 18 months. The irregular pigmentation and outline are very typical of a superficial spreading malignant melanoma.

Differential diagnosis of pigmented lesions

Mole (pigmented naevus)	Uniform colour
	Static or very slowly altering lesion (takes years)
	Even surface
Malignant melanoma	Irregular pigmentation or black
	Irregular surface
	Alteration in size occurs over weeks or months
	Erosion or appearance of surrounding pigmentation or satellite lesions are late signs
Seborrhoeic wart	Uniform light brown or occasionally darker shades
	Warty surface
	Has 'stuck-on' look
	Often multiple
Histiocytoma	Brownish firm lesion
	Mostly on limbs
Basal cell carcinoma	Nodular form is sometimes black or has flecks of pigment
	Mostly on face, but can occur elsewhere

pigmented lesions but these have to be distinguished from malignant melanoma, dermatofibroma, pigmented basal cell carcinoma (rodent ulcer) and angiomas of different types. Probably the greatest difficulty is experienced in identifying lesions that are suspected of being malignant melanoma. As already indicated, the diagnosis may be difficult and what follows must only be regarded as brief notes and hints on the topic. If there is any doubt the patient *must* be referred without delay to a specialist with experience of these lesions.

Diagnostic pointers

Moles As malignant melanoma may arise from an existing mole or from previously normal nonpigmented skin, the patient's statement as to what was previously at the site of the presenting lesion is not often much help. The following points may, however, be of use:

1. Ordinary moles gradually mature and later degenerate and disappear so that they become much less numerous in the elderly.
2. Inflammation in moles can be very difficult to distinguish from malignant melanoma. It is particularly common on the face in hairy moles whose hairs have been plucked; the mole enlarges suddenly, becomes red and tender, and may discharge.
3. Rapid increase in size and depth of colour in a pre-existing lesion must always be taken seriously.
4. Changes in the surface texture including erosion and crusting may be indicative of malignancy.
5. Pigmentation of surrounding skin and/or satellite nodules are also bad signs.

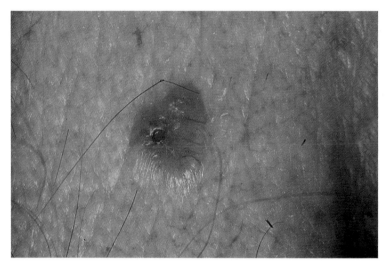

A pigmented nodular basal cell carcinoma. Sometimes these lesions can be much darker than this.

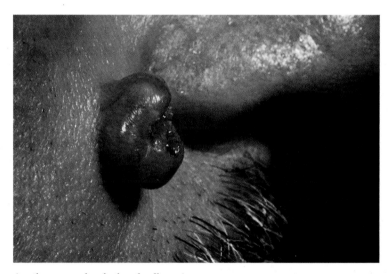

Another example of a basal cell carcinoma.

Seborrhoeic warts These develop on most people as they become older and are often misdiagnosed as malignant melanoma (see Chapter 26).

1. Their distinguishing feature is their wartiness which is not a feature of malignant melanoma.
2. Seborrhoeic warts don't usually occur singly.
3. They occur particularly over the chest, shoulders, back and face.

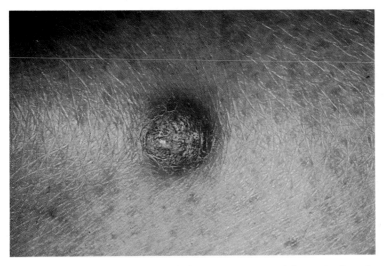

A typical histiocytoma. This firm, dark intercutaneous nodule occurred on the thigh of a 40-year-old woman and was confirmed histologically as a histiocytoma.

4. They often seem as if they are stuck on the skin surface or are plaque-like.
5. Their pigmentation is usually lighter than that of moles and is uniform.

Basal cell carcinoma This may be quite darkly pigmented – especially the nodular sort – and can confuse the unwary. They generally occur on the face and usually have the pearly sheen of ordinary basal cell carcinomas despite their pigmentation (see also Chapter 7).

Histiocytoma (dermatofibroma) This is a common type of fibrous nodule that mostly occurs on the limbs of middle-aged and elderly people. They are often pigmented (though not deeply) and are firm or even hard and seem deeply set in the skin. Occasionally they have a slightly warty and scaling surface. These lesions can also be confused with malignant melanoma.

VASCULAR MALFORMATIONS

Angioma

Another sort of skin lesion that can be quite difficult to distinguish is the small vascular malformation or angioma. The blood in these may suddenly clot and turn black, sometimes causing alarm in inexperienced doctors.

Pyogenic granuloma

A red, shiny or eroded nodule may suddenly appear which consists of a mass of young capillaries. These are inappropriately called pyogenic granulomas (inappropriately,

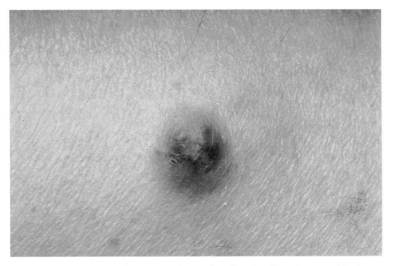

Angioma. Angiomatous lesions can be confused with other pigmented lesions, especially if they become clotted.

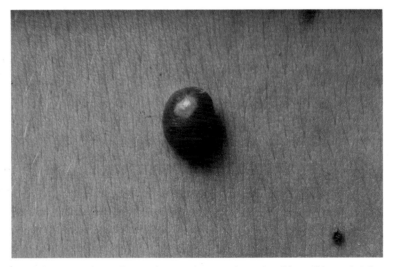

Typical pyogenic granuloma. This is projecting from the skin and has a bright red, glazed surface.

because they are neither pus-forming – pyogenic – nor due to granulomatous inflammation). Unfortunately malignant melanoma can look just like pyogenic granuloma especially if it is rapidly growing and nonpigmented.

WARTY LESIONS

When most people talk of warts they mean viral warts, and this is how I shall use the term here (see also Chapter 22). Warts are probably the commonest tumour of all; most of us have some warts at some stage and most disappear without specific treatment. The sites most often affected are the hand and fingers, the soles of the feet, the genitalia and the face – but they can occur virtually anywhere. Warts have different clinical appearances depending on the particular type of wart virus involved, the anatomical site infected and the resistance of the subject concerned:

1. On the hands viral warts are usually either proper warty nodules or small flat papules. The latter are either whitish-grey or pink and are known as plane warts.
2. On the soles, warts are either hard callous nodules or large plaques consisting of a mass of faceted papules (mosaic warts).
3. Warts on the face or on the genitalia often project straight out like horny spines or look like small cauliflowers. These are known as filiform warts.

Diagnostic problems

When large numbers of warts occur on the hand or feet of youngsters there is usually no difficulty in diagnosis. Some problems may arise in older subjects when the differentiation between viral warts, seborrhoeic warts (see pages 56–7), solar keratoses and even squamous cell carcinoma may be difficult. Squamous cell carcinoma should be suspected if the lesion is large and indurated. Hyperkeratotic warty and ulcerated types both occur.

Particular care should be taken with solitary warty lesions in elderly subjects. Although they may look like ordinary warts such lesions may actually be squamous cell carcinoma.

On the face, clusters of pink plane warts around the mouth and chin may look like acne or rosacea – such misdiagnoses are not as uncommon as you might think. Plane warts on the face tend to be uniform in appearance and not as inflamed as the lesions of acne and rosacea.

Solar keratoses

Solar keratoses (also called actinic and senile keratoses) are found in chronically sun-damaged skin (see also Chapter 11). They mostly occur on the backs of the hands and face but may also occur on the legs, the V of the neck or anywhere else that has been persistently exposed to the sun. They are recognized as pink or greyish-brown, raised, scaling or hyperkeratotic areas some 3–10 mm in diameter. Curious horny spines (cutaneous horns) may surmount these lesions. Solar keratoses, and indeed all types of solar damage, are more common in fair-complexioned blue-eyed folk, especially those of Celtic origin (see Chapter 11). A tiny proportion of these lesions eventually become frankly malignant although the exact proportion is uncertain. Their main importance is that they indicate that there has been a significant degree of solar damage and that a neoplastic lesion of some sort may develop at a site nearby.

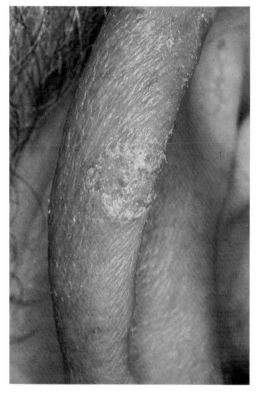

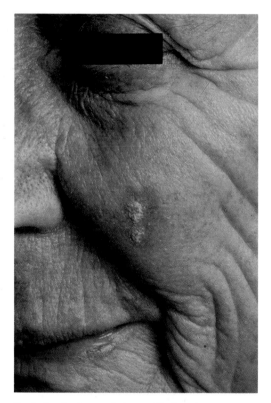

Scaling pink area on the external ear of an elderly patient, typical of a solar keratosis.

Typical solar keratosis in an elderly woman.

NODULES ON THE FACE

Basal cell carcinomas, senile sebaceous gland hyperplasia and nonpigmented moles can have a very similar clinical appearance.

Diagnostic pointers

Basal cell carcinoma This is a common slow-growing locally invasive neoplasm that occurs more commonly in light-exposed areas (see also Chapter 7). It is known colloquially as rodent ulcer. In the early stages the lesion is either a flat scaling macule or plaque or, more commonly, an opalescent or pearly nodule. These nodules often have flecks of pigment in them or may be more deeply and uniformly pigmented when they can be misdiagnosed as malignant melanoma (see page 218). Dilated blood vessels course over the surface of may of these lesions. When larger, the nodules ulcerate and form the then appropriately termed rodent ulcer.

Sebaceous gland hyperplasia This is a feature of facial skin in many elderly men. The reason for this curious benign localized hyperplastic response of sebaceous gland tissue is

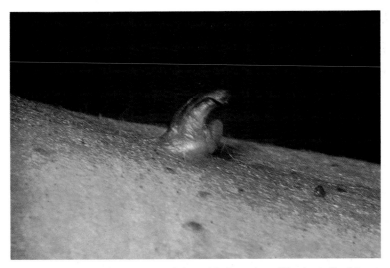

Cutaneous horn on the upper arm of an elderly patient. Histologically this was shown to have a solar keratosis in the base.

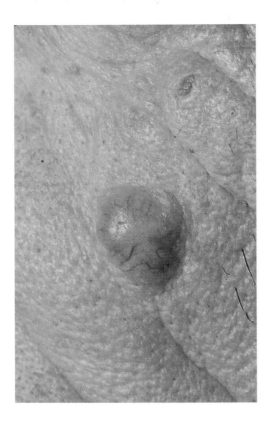

Typical cystic basal cell carcinoma occurring on the face of an elderly patient.

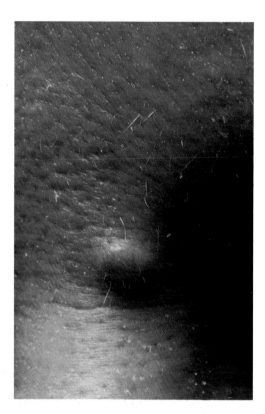

Nonpigmented mole on the bridge of the nose in a 37-year-old woman. This was misdiagnosed as a basal cell carcinoma.

obscure. The lesions are dome shaped, vary in colour from white to orangey-yellow and often have a central pit.

Nonpigmented moles Not all moles are pigmented and it is common to find that nodules removed from the face as rodent ulcers turn out to be simple moles when examined histologically. The surface of this type of nodule is sometimes loculated and may also have hairs sprouting from it.

Other nodules Other types of nodule are far less frequent on the face but there are several benign epithelial neoplasms that arise from hair follicles, such as trichoepithelioma and trichofolliculoma, which can cause confusion. In addition there are smaller nodules on the face including milia (which are really tiny epidermal cysts) and benign sweat gland tumours known as syringoma. The latter are whitish papules, 1–2 mm across, that occur symmetrically beneath the eyes and rarely much more extensively over the body. They are a cosmetic nuisance. Differentiation of all these lesions can be difficult – even for an expert. Adenoma sebaceum is, despite its name, neither an adenoma nor 'sebaceous'. It is the name for a benign fibrovascular tumour that usually occurs in large numbers on either side of the face paranasally. It is characteristic of a syndrome known as tuberous sclerosis in which central nervous system and other anomalies occur.

CYSTS

Acne cysts

Acne cysts contain pus and are not lined by an epithelium, and as such are not really cysts at all but cold abscesses. They are sometimes incorrectly called sebaceous cysts. They are characteristic of severe acne.

Epidermoid cysts

These contain keratinous debris and can occur anywhere, although they are most common on the face or trunk. They vary in size and not infrequently become inflamed.

Pilar cysts

Pilar cysts are formed by a particular part of the follicular epithelium and contain a special kind of horn (trichilemmal horn) found in the hair follicle. They occur over the scalp (especially in women) sometimes in large numbers, and also over the scrotum. They may be inherited as an autosomal dominant characteristic.

Sebaceous cysts

The only true sebaceous cyst is a rare congenital cystic lesion which contains sebum and is termed sebocystoma multiplex (multiplex – because several lesions occur together). These lesions are lined by sebaceous gland epithelium and are the only source of pure sebum. The lesions are usually small skin-coloured cysts, and occur on the trunk or face.

Dermoid cysts

These are uncommon congenital cysts that occur around the orbit and need skilled surgical treatment.

PRACTICAL POINTS

- Diagnostic problems with skin tumours are common, often difficult to solve and extremely important in terms of outcome.
- Lesions that may be confused with malignant melanoma include:
  –Moles
  –Seborrhoeic warts
  –Histiocytoma
  –Angioma
  –Pyogenic granuloma.
- If there is any doubt about diagnosis in the above conditions immediate specialist advice is essential.
- Solitary warty lesions in the elderly may be squamous cell carcinoma.

37

Pointers to systemic disease

BACKGROUND

Some skin disorders point to serious internal disease and need to be recognized quickly. It is not appropriate to describe every one of these conditions here, but I will point out some of the most important of them so that some idea can be gained of the range of associations between disease of skin and visceral disorders.

SKIN CONDITIONS THAT INDICATE SYSTEMIC DISEASE

Erythema nodosum

This is characterized by tender red nodules which occur suddenly over the shins accompanied by general malaise and fever, and may signal the presence of visceral tuberculosis or sarcoidosis. It can also be a complication of ulcerative colitis and Crohn's disease, drug intake (sulphonamides) and some types of viral infection.

Erythema multiforme

Erythema multiforme often occurs spontaneously without an identifiable precipitating cause, but it also occurs subsequent to herpes simplex and other types of infection. It can also be provoked by drugs – sulphonamides and hydantoinates, for example (see Chapter 13).

Acquired ichthyosis

The sudden onset of dryness and scaliness of the skin surface can be a sign of underlying visceral malignant disease – the reticuloses in particular. It may also be seen in association with intestinal malabsorption.

Pigmentation

A generalized increase in skin pigmentation may be seen in Addison's disease, visceral malignancy and coeliac disease. Less commonly it can be due to the administration of certain drugs – chlorpromazine (Largactil) and compounds containing silver.

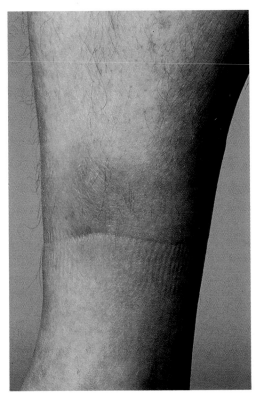 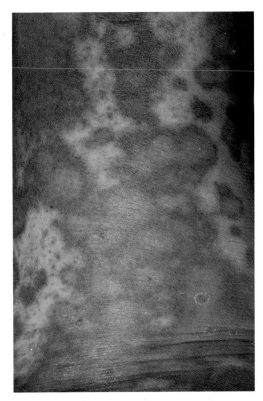

Erythema nodosum. A very tender dusky red area on the shin of a 28-year-old woman later found to have sarcoidosis.

Severe erythroderma multiforme. Some target-type lesions are seen. This patient was quite sick with her skin complaint. The mouth was extensively eroded and the eyes showed some conjunctivitis.

Acanthosis nigricans

This rare condition causes darkening and thickening of the skin of the flexures, and thickening of palmar skin and buccal mucosa. When present it may signify a gastrointestinal adenocarcinoma or other type of visceral malignancy, though it is also a complication of certain types of pituitary disorder.

Dermatomyositis

An inflammatory disorder of skin and muscle of the auto-immune type with similarities to lupus erythematosus (see pages 78 and 166). Its presence may rarely signify a visceral malignancy – particularly of the genital tract in women, and carcinoma of the bronchus or breast.

Pemphigoid

May also be a skin marker of neoplastic disease, although this is not the case in most patients with this disorder.

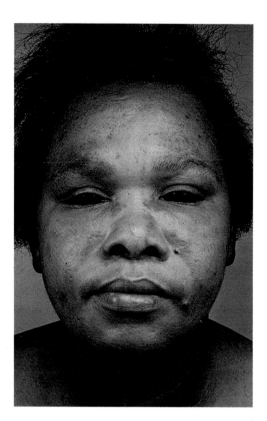

Dermatomyositis. There is swelling around the eyes and some dusky erythema. This woman felt generally unwell and had tender weak limb girdle muscles.

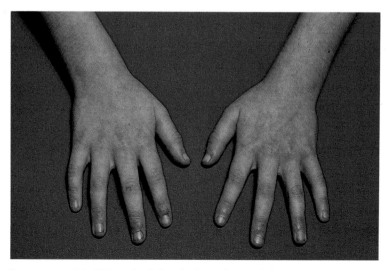

Dermatomyositis. This patient's hands showed typical changes over the skin of the fingers with redness and involvement of the skin over the extensor aspects of the joints.

Urticaria

Sometimes indicative of serious systemic diseases such an anaphylactoid purpura and lupus erythematosus (see Chapter 34).

Generalized itchiness

Can be caused by jaundice, renal failure, polycythaemia rubra vera, disorders of calcium metabolism and the reticuloses (see Chapter 17).

SYSTEMIC DISEASES ACCOMPANIED BY SKIN DISORDERS

Virilizing syndromes

These can be indicated by the onset or worsening of acne, increased hair growth on the limbs and trunk, and bitemporal recession of the scalp hair margin in women (see Chapter 24).

Cushing's syndrome

Livid striae over the upper arms, thighs and abdomen may indicate hypercortisonism resulting from either Cushing's syndrome or from steroid administration. A beefy red complexion, acne and pads of fat over the supraclavicular and cervical regions are also present in Cushing's syndrome.

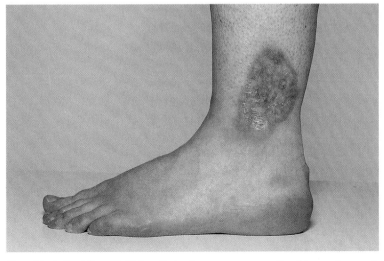

Necrobiosis lipoidica. Pinkish yellow plaques occur over the shins and around the ankles in this disorder. In this patient the skin showed some atrophic change and as usual the condition was very resistant to all forms of treatment.

Diabetes

In diabetes an odd skin condition known as necrobiosis lipoidica diabeticorum may develop over the shins. The lesions are circumscribed, irregularly raised pinkish-yellow plaques that tend to persist for very long periods of time.

Perigenital candidiasis may also be seen in diabetes but a tendency to develop boils and abscesses is much less frequent than often stated. Generalized itchiness as a sign of diabetes also is more myth than reality.

PRACTICAL POINTS

Skin markers of malignancy:

- **Acanthosis nigricans**
  –Thickening, wartiness and increased pigmentation of flexural areas
  –May also be thickening on palms and on buccal mucosa
  –Rare
  –Occurs mostly in association with adenocarcinomata.
- **Dermatomyositis**
  –Reddened areas over face, fingers and elsewhere in association with proximal muscle tenderness and weakness
  –Mostly *not* an association of malignancy but has been noted in carcinoma of the bronchus and in women with genital tract cancers and carcinoma of the breast.
- **Pemphigoid**
  –Blistering disorder
  –May rarely indicate an underlying malignancy.
- **Acquired ichthyosis**
  –Sudden onset of generalized scaling in mature life may indicate underlying reticulosis or more commonly other types of neoplasia.
- **Necrolytic migratory erythema**
  –Rare progressive erosive erythematous rash often indicating a tumour of alpha cells of the pancreas.
- **Annular erythemas**
  –One type in particular in which there are concentric erythematous rings (erythema gyratum perstans) usually signifies the presence of a neoplasm.
- **Cutaneous metastases**
  –Nodules, papules and plaques due to metastasis occur in 5–10 per cent of patients with carcinomatosis
  –Lung, breast, prostate and stomach are common primary sites.

38

Appropriate investigations

Most of the investigations required for diagnosis of common skin disorders have already been mentioned but they have been grouped together in this final chapter for easy reference. Most of these should only be performed by specialists; however, the practitioner will be responsible for subsequent management of the patient and so must have an understanding of what the tests involve.

SKIN SCRAPINGS FOR RINGWORM

It is often quite difficult to decide whether a rash is due to a ringworm fungus or not (see Chapter 31). The site should be investigated for the presence of the micro-organism *before* any treatment is prescribed. It may be necessary to repeat the investigation two or three times before it is absolutely certain whether ringworm is present or not.

The area of affected skin is gently scraped with a blunt scalpel and the resulting scales are placed either in a plain envelope or between two glass slides which are then bound together. The specimens are sent to the local mycology laboratory, where they will be examined both by direct microscopy and by culture techniques. The results of culture may take several weeks to arrive back, as fungi affecting the skin grow slowly. Before sending off the specimens to a laboratory it is best to make personal contact with the pathologist in charge to ensure that the specimens are taken in the best way for the particular laboratory and that the laboratory is geared to the particular investigation.

PATCH TESTING

Patch testing is designed to determine whether a patient has an allergic contact hypersensitivity and should only be performed when the patient has dermatitis (see Chapters 15 and 34). It is not an appropriate investigation for urticaria or other types of hypersensitivity. It can generate extremely important information, but if done incorrectly can cause great confusion. For this reason it should be carried out by experienced staff in a department of dermatology. Patients with active dermatitis are not usually investigated by patch testing until the rash has quietened down, as patch testing can provoke quite a bad flaring of the condition. The tests require at least three visits to the clinic and the patient should be warned about this. The allergens (often a series or 'battery' of allergens is used) are placed in contact with the skin (usually the back) with specially

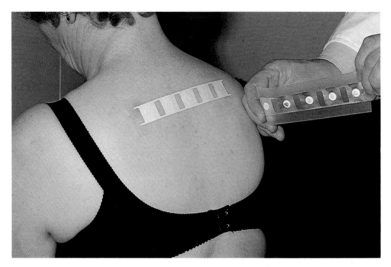

Patch tests being applied. The materials applied on the patches are those that commonly sensitize. In most test batteries about 20 such patches are placed on the back and left in position for 48 hours.

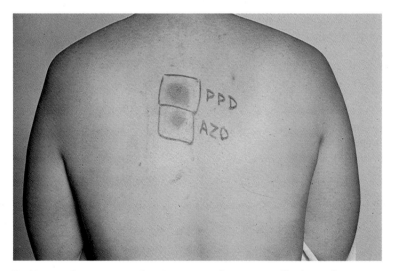

Positive patch tests to two dyes in a patient known to suffer from allergic contact dermatitis due to dyes. Paraphenylenediamine (PPD) is a frequently used blue-black dye. AZO stands for a group of dyes commonly used to give red and yellow colours. The patches have been left in place for 48 hours.

designed adhesive dressings and kept in place for 48 hours. They are then removed and read. They are examined again after a further 24 or 48 hours to pick up any late reactors.

A positive test doesn't necessarily indicate that the particular allergen is responsible for the patient's rash. It may just signify that he or she possesses that particular

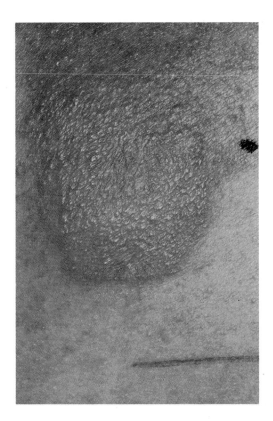

A positive patch test result. The skin is swollen, reddened and surmounted by many small vesicles.

hypersensitivity. Each test has to be interpreted in the light of the particular subject's history and rash. Care must also be taken to exclude false positives from simple irritation by the material or the dressing.

Sometimes the patient is tested with the actual suspected substance under occlusion. Or the patient can perform a 'use' test with a suspected article or substance so that the actual circumstances of exposure are reproduced. This test is performed without an occlusive dressing. In this case care has to be taken to ensure that the substance is not merely irritant, causing a false positive.

SCRATCH, PRICK AND INTRACUTANEOUS TESTS

When a patient has urticaria or an allergy of the immediate type these tests may give important information as to the allergen responsible. They are also used in some patients with atopy to determine whether they have particular hypersensitivities.

The allergens are specially made-up solutions and once again, the tests should be done in an experienced department because not only is the technique of the testing procedure important, but the interpretation can be extremely tricky. In addition, if a drug hypersensitivity is suspected (as with penicillin) there is the danger that the patient might go into anaphylactic shock, and all facilities for resuscitation should be present at the place of testing.

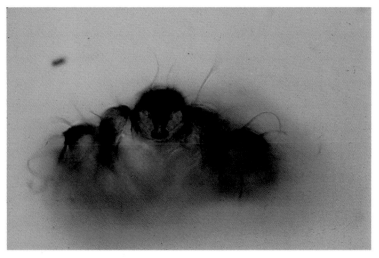

A scabies mite as seen when removed by taking off a strip of the horny layer with a rapidly bonding glue – a technique called skin surface biopsy.

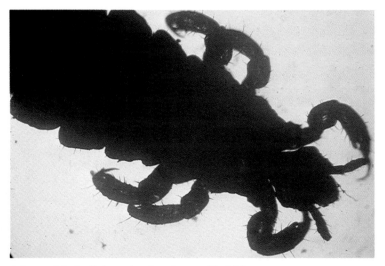

A louse picked off the scalp of an 8-year-old child.

PHOTO TESTING

Patients with rashes in the light-exposed areas (see Chapter 11) may require special tests to determine whether they have a hypersensitivity to sunlight. These tests can be complex and require special apparatus (a monochromator) as it may be necessary to test to particular wavelengths of sunlight. There are few centres in the UK that can perform these tests so the patient may need to travel long distances to reach a suitable centre. It

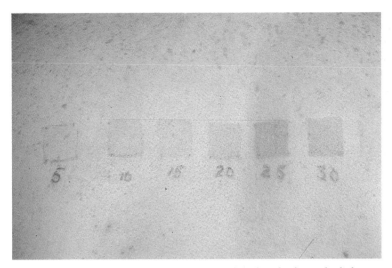

Small areas of skin on the back have been irradiated with ultraviolet light from a sun-lamp for different periods of time to obtain the minimum dose (in seconds) at which persistent erythema remains after 8 hours. This is called the minimal erythema dose.

may also be necessary to test the patients to light after application of materials that can cause photosensitization. This procedure is known as photopatch testing.

IDENTIFICATION OF MITES, LICE AND BITING INSECTS

It is not always easy to identify insect bites or determine whether a rash is due to scabies or not. Sometimes a visit to the home is helpful to seek out the biting insect. It may also be necessary to brush out the coat of pets and take the brushings to a veterinarian to identify the presence of eggs and insect remains. It is quite a skilful task to dig out a scabies mite from her burrow for identification, so unless your eyesight is very good and you have plenty of time, leave it to the dermatologist!

Epilogue

Skin disease is, in general, poorly taught in medical schools. Because it doesn't possess the high drama of other specialties it has not been allotted its rightful place either in the allocation of teaching time or in the provision of resources. I find that practitioners hunger after some dermatological know-how. They recognize the importance of skin disease in the community even if their peers in medical school don't! I hope that this book has been of some assistance to them. In its essentially practical approach I have tried to outline the common problems and what to do when they are encountered.

The only way that skin disease differs from disease of other systems is that its signs and progress are easily visible. This should not dictate any difference in approach. Diagnosis comes before treatment; treatment includes general management as well as the prescription of ointments and creams. If, after reading about the various problems I have included, the reader feels better equipped to deal with them, my efforts will have been rewarded.

Useful addresses

British Red Cross
Beauty Care and Cosmetic Camouflage Section
9 Grosvenor Crescent
London SW1X 7EG
(Tel 0171 235 5454)

British Association of Dermatologists
19 Fitzroy Square
London W1
(Tel 0171 383 0266)

Cancer Information Service
3 Bath Place
London EC2 3JR
(Tel 0171 613 2121)

Cancer Research Campaign
6–10 Cambridge Terrace
London NW1 4JL
(Tel 0171 224 1333)

D.E.B.R.A. (Dystrophic Epidermolysis Bullosa Research Association)
D.E.B.R.A. House
13 Wellington Business Park
Duke's Ride
Crowthorne
Berks RG11 6LS
(Tel 01344 771961)

Imperial Cancer Research Fund
44 Lincolns Inn Fields
London WC2A 3PX
(Tel 0171 242 0200)

Lupus Group
Olivier Hanscombe
18 Stephenson Way
London NW1 2HD
(Tel 0171 916 1500)

M.A.R.C.S. (Melanoma and Related Cancers of the Skin)
Dermatology Treatment Centre
Level 3
Salisbury District Hospital
Salisbury
Wilts
(Tel 01722 415071)

National Eczema Society
163 Eversholt Street
London NW1 1HT
(Tel 0171 388 4097)

Psoriasis Association
7 Milton Street
Northampton NN2 7JG
(Tel 01604 711129)

S.C.A.R. (Skin Charity to Advance Research)
Department of Medicine (Dermatology)
University of Wales College of Medicine
Heath Park
Cardiff CF4 4XN
(Tel 01222 747747)

Bibliography

Champion RH. Psoriasis and its treatment. *British Medical Journal* 1981; **282**: 343–6.

Cunliffe WJ, Cotterill JA. *The Acnes*. London: WB Saunders Co, 1975.

Cronin E. *Contact Dermatitis*. Edinburgh: Churchill Livingstone, 1980.

Farber EM, Cox AJ, eds. *Psoriasis*. New York: Grune and Stratton, 1982.

Hall-Smith P, Cairns RJ. *Dermatology: Current Concepts and Practice*. London: Butterworth-Heinemann, 1981.

MacKie RM. *Clinical Dermatology* 3rd edn. Oxford: Oxford University Press, 1991.

MacKie RM, Rowell NR, eds. Skin disorders. *Medicine International 1 & 2* 1983: Parts 27 & 28.

Magnus IA. *Dermatological Photobiology*. Oxford: Blackwell Scientific Publications, 1976.

Marks R, Christophers E, eds. *The Epidermis in Disease*. Lancaster: MTP Press, 1981.

Marks R, Dykes PJ, eds. *The Icthyoses*. Lancaster: MTP Press, 1978.

Marks R, Plewig G, eds. *Stratum Corneum*. Heidelberg: Springer-Verlag, 1983.

Rajka G. *Atopic Dermatitis*. London: WB Saunders Co, 1975.

Shuster S. *Dermatology in Internal Medicine*. Oxford: Oxford University Press, 1978.

Acknowledgements

I thank Professor R Moreton and the Department of Medical Illustration of the University Hospital of Wales for their considerable help in obtaining most of the illustrations for this book. Thanks are also due to the Department of Paediatrics of the University of Wales College of Medicine for some of the illustrations, and to Dr Richard Staughton and the Photographic Department of Westminster Medical School for supplying the photograph on page 14 (right hand side).

I would also like to record my sincere thanks to my secretarial staff who prepared the manuscript and to my registrars who put up with my ill-humour during its preparation.

Ronald Marks 1996

Index